COPD
COPD

David MG Halpin MA, DPhil (OXON), MB BS (LOND), FRCP

Consultant Physician and Senior Lecturer in Respiratory Medicine
Royal Devon and Exeter Hospital, Exeter, UK

MOSBY
An affiliate of Elsevier Science Limited

ISBN 0-7234-3268-6

First published 2001
Reprinted 2002

Cataloguing in Publication Data
Catalogue records for this book are available from the US Library of Congress and the British Library.

Note
Medical knowledge is constantly changing. As new information becomes available, changes in treatment, procedures, equipment and the use of drugs become necessary. The authors and publishers have, as far as it is possible, taken care to ensure that the information given in this text is accurate and up to date. However, readers are strongly advised to confirm that the information, especially with regard to drug usage, complies with latest legislation and standards of practice.

your source for books,
journals and multimedia
in the health sciences

www.elsevierhealth.com

The
publisher's
policy is to use
**paper manufactured
from sustainable forests**

Printed by Grafos

Acknowledgements

This book could not have been written without the support, encouragement and understanding of Helen, Philippa and Isabelle. I am grateful to friends and colleagues for comments on the manuscripts but any errors or omissions remain entirely my responsibility.

Foreword

Respiratory problems have a special place in medical care because in many western countries they form the largest single reason for patients consulting doctors.

For acute conditions the challenge for primary care is how to manage large numbers of patients, most of whom will not have major pathology, whilst swiftly and skilfully identifying any one of whom who may have serious pathology, whether tuberculosis, cancer or even malaria or meningitis which can present as "flu".

For chronic respiratory diseases, the dominant conditions are asthma and chronic obstructive pulmonary disease. As many as ten per cent of the whole population in some places may have one of these, so that big numbers of patients and consultations are involved. With the advent of new medications and better research much more is now known about how to optimise care. The keys are sensitive listening and appropriate explanations, with the professional building a sustained partnership with the patient over time to help them maintain modern treatment regimes.

What constitutes up-to-date treatment is therefore always an issue. This new book integrates perspectives from both primary and secondary care and provides practical, evidence-based guidance on care.

Sir Denis Pereira Gray OBE, MA, HonDSc,
FRCP, FRCGP, HonFFPHM, FMedSci
Institute of General Practice/SaNDNet
University of Exeter
October 2001

Contents

Introduction and Background

Chronic obstructive pulmonary disease (COPD) is one of the most common chronic diseases in the UK. It is a major cause of morbidity and mortality, but it is often forgotten that it is preventable. In less than 20 years it will be one of the five leading medical burdens on society worldwide.[1] It results in around 30,000 deaths annually in the UK, just over one in 20 of all deaths. It results in frequent consultation in primary care and considerable use of hospital services, accounting for around 10% of all medical admissions. On average, a GP will have at least 200 patients with COPD. Each year around 50 will consult their GP, 20 will have acute exacerbations, five will be admitted to hospital and one or two will die.

Many patients are unaware that they have a chronic disease and expect simple, one-off treatments to cure their symptoms. The majority of patients will only present at the time of an exacerbation and will not be part of a chronic disease management programme. Their management in primary care is challenging, not least because they continue to have symptoms despite treatment and follow an inexorable downward course. Patients with COPD have often been seen as "heart-sink" patients with a self-inflicted condition for whom little therapy is available. In fact, although most current treatments do not affect disease progression, symptomatic relief can produce marked improvements in patients' quality of life.

As with asthma, the organization of care is vitally important. Although structured care for patients with COPD is only just being introduced, there is evidence that it reduces emergency consultations, improves patients' understanding of their disease and their ability to self-manage, and gives an opportunity to rationalize therapy and identify complications.

Terminology

Chronic obstructive pulmonary disease (COPD) is now the preferred designation[2] for a group of conditions variously known as chronic airflow limitation (CAL), chronic obstructive airways disease (COAD), chronic obstructive lung disease (COLD), chronic bronchitis and emphysema. The term COPD was coined in the early 1960s and is preferred because it encapsulates the fact that the condition not only affects the airways, but also affects the lung parenchyma and the pulmonary circulation. However, many patients and some doctors still do not recognize or use the term and persist with the older terminology.

Classical descriptions of chronic bronchitis and emphysema were made in the early nineteenth century, but modern interest in the condition did not begin until many patients died during the London smogs of the late 1950s.[3] Around this time, spirometry was becoming available and this led to the observation that airflow obstruction was the key factor in determining disability and mortality.[4] These studies, and confusion about the best terminology to use in epidemiological studies, led to the 1958 CIBA symposium which suggested definitions of chronic bronchitis, emphysema, and variable and fixed airflow obstruction.[5] Emphysema was defined in anatomical terms, whilst chronic bronchitis was defined clinically as "chronic or recurrent excessive mucus secretion in the bronchial tree". The introduction of the physiological concept of airflow limitation as a diagnostic term was new.

The epidemiology, causation and natural history of COPD have been extensively studied over the last 40 years, but some questions still remain unanswered. Interest in COPD has increased again recently, partly as a result of the publication of clinical guidelines on its management, but also in recognition of its prevalence and the significant morbidity and mortality it causes.

Definition and Epidemiology

COPD is a chronic, slowly progressive disease characterized by airflow obstruction that shows minimal diurnal or day-to-day variation. Variability of airflow limitation is not dichotomous and in practice there is a spectrum of reversibility (Figures 1 and 2).

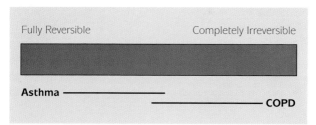

Figure 1. The spectrum of reversibility of airflow obstruction in COPD and asthma.

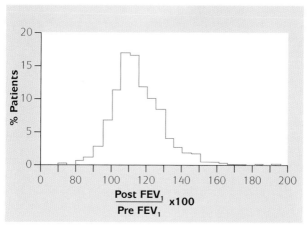

Figure 2. Frequency distribution of bronchodilator reversibility in patients with COPD. Reproduced with permission from Anthonisen NR *et al.* Bronchodilator response in chronic obstructive pulmonary disease. *Am Rev Respir Disease* 1986; **133**: 814–819.[6]

Definition

The original description of COPD emphasized the obstruction to airflow, especially on expiration, its large irreversible component and tendency to progress. Chronic bronchitis and emphysema are specific conditions with distinct clinical or pathological features, but there is considerable overlap with COPD. There may also be some overlap with asthma, which if long-standing and poorly treated can lead to irreversible airflow limitation. COPD may also develop in asthmatics who smoke and the two conditions may co-exist. Some patients with COPD have partially reversible airflow limitation and this is often referred to as an "asthmatic component" (Table 1).

Definitions of COPD
British Thoracic Society[2]
A chronic, slowly progressive disorder characterized by airflow obstruction (reduced FEV_1 and FEV_1/VC ratio) that does not change markedly over several months. Most of the lung function impairment is fixed, although some reversibility can be produced by bronchodilator (or other) therapy.
American Thoracic Society[7]
COPD is a disease state characterized by the presence of airflow obstruction due to chronic bronchitis or emphysema; the airflow obstruction is generally progressive, may be accompanied by airway hyperreactivity, and may be partially reversible.
European Respiratory Society[8]
COPD is disorder characterized by reduced maximum expiratory flow and slow forced emptying of the lungs; features which do not change markedly over several months. Most of the airflow limitation is slowly progressive and irreversible. The airflow limitation is due to varying combinations of airways disease and emphysema; the relative contribution of the two processes is difficult to define *in vivo*.
GOLD[9]
COPD is a disease state characterized by airflow limitation that is not fully reversible. The airflow limitation is usually both progressive and associated with an abnormal inflammatory response of the lungs to noxious particles or gases

Table 1. Definitions of COPD.

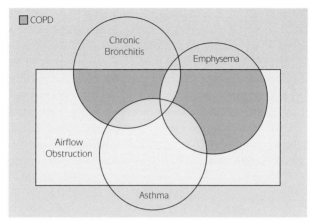

Figure 3. Venn diagram illustrating the overlap between the diagnoses of chronic bronchitis, emphysema and asthma, and their contribution to COPD.

The overlap with asthma remains an everyday clinical problem and when defined according to the degree of reversible airflow limitation, the boundary is to a certain extent arbitrary, particularly as it is increasingly recognized that the degree of reversibility in individual patients may vary from day to day (Figure 3). There are differences in the profile of inflammatory cells present in the airways of patients with asthma and COPD, but these are not amenable to routine clinical measurement.

Other lung diseases, such as bronchiectasis or obliterative bronchiolitis, may cause substantially irreversible airflow limitation or chronic mucus secretion, but these are not generally included as part of the spectrum of COPD. Bronchopulmonary dysplasia, which occurs as a result of neonatal mechanical ventilation,[10] is a cause of irreversible airflow obstruction and as more of these children are now reaching middle age, it may become an increasing cause of diagnostic confusion with COPD.

Aetiology

The aetiology of COPD is multi-factorial, but in western countries cigarette smoking is unquestionably the major aetiological factor. It accounts for approximately 80% of the attributable risk.[11] There is a clear dose–response relationship between total tobacco consumption and the risk of developing COPD, as well as the severity of the disease; however, not all smokers will develop COPD and susceptibility factors, possibly genetic, are also important.

In 1976, Fletcher and colleagues published their landmark study of the natural history of airflow obstruction in COPD.[12] The key features were the more rapid loss of lung function in a proportion of smokers, the wide differences in susceptibility to developing obstruction between smokers, and the effects of quitting smoking in slowing the annual decline in FEV$_1$ (forced expiratory volume in 1 second). The airflow limitation due to smoking developed gradually, even in susceptible individuals, and patients had airflow limitation for many years before becoming symptomatic (Figure 4).

It is now realized that smoking may lead to the development of COPD by (a) reducing the maximum lung function that is attained, (b) leading to an earlier onset of decline in lung function, (c) leading to an accelerated rate of decline, or (d) a combination of these (Figure 5).

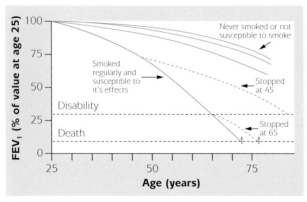

Figure 4. Natural history of COPD as proposed by Fletcher and Peto. Reproduced with permission from Fletcher C, Peto R. The natural history of chronic airflow obstruction. *Br Med J* 1977; **1** (6077): 1645–1648. Copyright © 1977 BMJ Publishing Group.[13]

Although the median FEV_1 falls as cigarette consumption increases and a tail of low values develops, FEV_1 can be normal despite heavy cigarette consumption[14] (Figure 6). On the basis of Fletcher and Peto's work, the proportion of smokers thought to be susceptible to smoking is often quoted as being around 20%. This overlooks early mortality of smokers, and if this is taken into account the proportion may be much higher.

Differences in cigarette smoking only account for around 15% of the variation in lung function,[15] but it is still not known which factors influence an individual smoker's susceptibility to developing airflow obstruction. Family[16] and twin[17] studies have shown that COPD genetic factors are important, but the effects are complex.[18]

Alpha-1 antitrypsin (α-1 AT) deficiency is the only known genetic risk factor for COPD, but it accounts for only about 2% of cases of severe COPD. It is associated with the development of emphysema in non-smokers, but the risk is substantially higher in smokers (see below). Extensive studies are underway to try to identify other genetic risk factors.[19]

The damage caused by smoking is cumulative and thus a second major risk factor for COPD is age. Most patients present in their fifth or sixth decade, by which time they have smoked for 20–30 years.

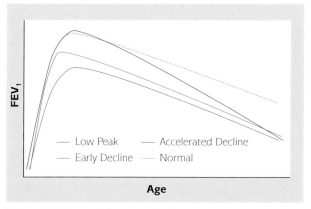

Figure 5. Schema of the range of effects of smoking on the age-related changes in lung function.

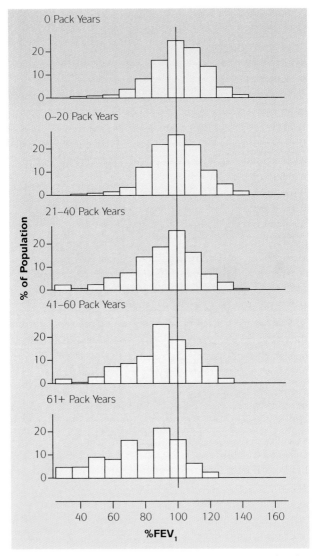

Figure 6. Range of lung function seen in smokers. Reproduced with permission from Burrows *et al.* Quantitative relationships between cigarette smoking and ventilatory function. *Am Rev Respir Dis* 1977; **115**(2): 195–205.[14]

In addition to smoking, two other risk factors have been proposed: recurrent bronchopulmonary infections (the so-called "British hypothesis"); and pre-existing atopy and airway hyperresponsiveness (the so-called "Dutch hypothesis").[20] There is evidence to support a role for each of these.

Early studies could not show an effect of recurrent infections in accelerating decline in the relatively healthy smokers.[21,22] However, once airflow obstruction has developed, mucus hypersecretion and/or infections may lead to further accelerated decline in lung function.[23-26] Recent work has also shown that patients with established COPD can be split into those with infrequent exacerbations (less than two per year) and those with frequent exacerbations (three or more per year).[27] The lung function of patients having frequent exacerbations often does not recover to the pre-exacerbation level before the next exacerbation occurs, leading to progressive decline.

The effects of cigarette smoking on the rate of decline in FEV_1 are greater in the presence of airway hyper-responsiveness.[28]

Prior to the marked increase in tobacco consumption in the UK in the late nineteenth century, environmental factors appear to have been the most important causes of what would now be called COPD, and this may remain the case worldwide.[29] In the UK, environmental factors and occupational dust exposures, particularly in coal miners,[30] are still important in some cases. Occupational dust exposures can cause cough and sputum production, which could be considered as bronchitis, but many of these patients do not have significant airflow obstruction and there is no loss of elastic recoil or evidence of emphysema. These patients do not, therefore, have COPD. Some occupational exposures are, however, associated with the development of COPD. The most well characterized are: cotton dust; grain dust; cement dust; oil fumes; and cadmium fumes.[31,32]

The incidence of COPD has always had a strong socio-economic bias and this persisted even in the years when cigarette smoking was relatively evenly distributed across socio-

Risk Factors for COPD
Cigarette smoking
Age
Dusty occupation
Environmental pollution
α-1 AT deficiency
Low birthweight
Frequent childhood infections
Damp housing
Diet low in dark fish, fruit and antioxidants

Table 2. Risk factors for COPD.

economic groups. Low birthweight and frequent childhood infections have been associated with an increased risk of COPD[33,34] and this may partly explain the link with low socio-economic status. Similarly, damp housing and a diet low in fish, fruit and vegetables containing antioxidants, are associated with an increased risk of COPD,[35,36] and these factors may also explain the link with poor socio-economic status (Table 2).

α-1 Antitrypsin deficiency

α-1 Antitrypsin (or α-1 antiprotease) is the major protease inhibitor in serum and in the lungs. It protects tissues against enzymatic digestion by several enzymes released by activated neutrophils, including neutrophil elastase.[37] In 1963, α-1 AT deficiency was first identified and it was recognized to be associated with the early onset of severe lower zone emphysema.[38] α-1 AT deficiency accounts for around 2% of cases of COPD.

The enzymes inhibited by α-1 AT have been shown to be capable of producing emphysema in experimental models, and so it has been suggested that in patients with α-1 AT deficiency there is excessive, unopposed activity of neutrophil proteases with consequent lung damage (Figure 7). α-1 AT deficiency is also associated with cirrhosis, primary hepatocellular carcinoma and systemic vasculitis (Table 3).[39]

The two common forms of α-1 AT deficiency result from point mutations in the gene that codes for α-1 AT (Figure 8). These are known as S and Z on the basis of the electrophoretic

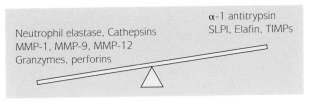

Figure 7. The normal balance between proteases and antiproteases.

Clinical Manifestations of α-1 antitrypsin deficiency
Early onset emphysema Hepatic cirrhosis Hepatocellular carcinoma Systemic Vasculitis

Table 3. Clinical manifestations of α-1 AT deficiency.

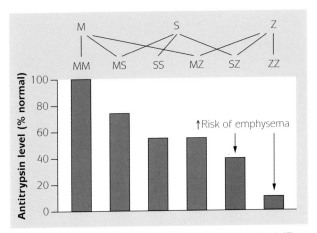

Figure 8. Relationship between α-1 AT phenotype and α-1 AT levels.

mobility of the protein they produce. The normal allele is known as M. The ZZ genotype results in α-1 AT levels around 10% of normal, whilst MZ heterozygotes have levels around 55% normal. SS homozygotes also have levels around 55% normal and MS heterozygotes have levels around 75% normal. The SZ genotype is associated with α-1 AT levels around 40% normal.[40] The development of emphysema is associated with deficiency of the ZZ phenotype[41] and severe deficiency of the SZ phenotype,[42] as well as with the rarer null phenotypes.[43] However, not all patients with the ZZ genotype develop emphysema, even if they are smokers.[44]

There are marked geographical variations in the prevalence of the genes for the S and M types of α-1 AT in Europe (Figure 9). The Z allele is rare in Black and Asian populations. The S allele is commonest in Spain and Portugal, and the Z allele is commonest in countries bordering the North Sea.[45] In the UK, the overall gene frequencies for the S and Z alleles are around 4.5% and 2% respectively, giving a ZZ homozygote prevalence of around one in 2,500.

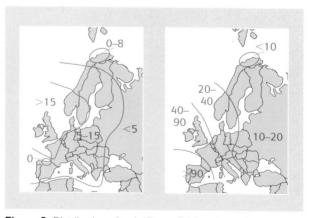

Figure 9. Distribution of α-1 AT type Z (a) and type S (b) genes in Europe. Reproduced from Hutchison DC. Alpha1-Proteinase inhibitor deficiency. In: Brewis RAL, Corrin B, Geddes DM, Gibson GJ, editors. *Respiratory Medicine*. London: W. B. Saunders, 1995; pp. 1034–1041.[46]

There is considerable variability in the clinical manifestations of patients with α-1 AT deficiency, with some patients having minimal or no symptoms and others developing severe emphysema at an early age. Smoking is the major factor influencing the development of emphysema, but some non-smokers develop airflow limitation in later life and this appears to be associated with a history of asthma or pneumonia.[39]

Epidemiology

COPD is an important cause of death worldwide, but there are significant variations in the age-standardized mortality rates between countries (Figure 10).

COPD accounts for over 25,000 deaths in England and Wales each year,[47] but the burden of disease is considerably greater. Morbidity from COPD is high, and patients are frequent users of primary and secondary care facilities. As many as one in eight hospital admissions may be due to COPD and consultation rates in General Practice are at least twice as high

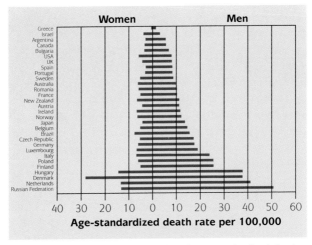

Figure 10. Comparison of international age-standardized death rates from COPD (based on data from the World Health Organization).

as those for angina.[48] They rise with age from 417 per year per 1,000 patients aged 45–64 to 1,032 per year per 1,000 patients aged 75–84.[49] The cost to the economy is also high, with an estimated 27 million working days lost per year.

It is difficult to be sure how common COPD is because many patients with mild disease are not diagnosed and do not consult their doctors. Surveys based on questionnaires cannot identify patients with airflow limitation and there is only one national study measuring airway function in patients aged 18–65 in the UK. Overall, 10% of men and 11% of women had an abnormally low FEV_1.[50] In the primary care population in the UK, the prevalence of an abnormal FEV_1 and respiratory symptoms was around 9%.[51] In the USA, the prevalence of physician diagnosed emphysema or abnormal lung function was 4–6% in white males and 1–3% in white females.[52] In black populations in the USA, the prevalence of a low FEV_1 was 3.7% in men and 6.7% in women.[53] The prevalence increases with increasing age.

It is also difficult to be certain of the true mortality due to COPD. Some patients will die with the disease rather than because of it and others will die of causes related to COPD, but their death may be certified as being due to these complications.[54] Analysis of trends in death rates is also complicated by changes in the diagnostic labels. The latest figures suggest that there were 27,932 deaths due to COPD in the UK in 1999.[47] This represents 5.1% of all deaths (4.3% of all male deaths and 5.9% of all female deaths). In men, age-standardized mortality rates from COPD have fallen progressively over the last 30 years, but in women there has been a small but progressive increase over the last 20 years[55] (Figure 11, Table 4).

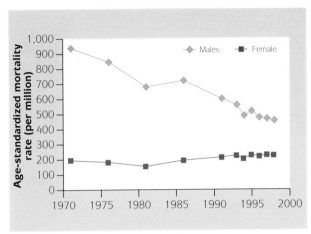

Figure 11. Trends in male and female age-standardized mortality rates from COPD in England and Wales between 1970 and 1998.

Epidemiology of COPD in England and Wales

Approximately 25,000 deaths per year
4.3% of male and 5.9% of female deaths
Prevalence of COPD approximately 10% in adults over 45
Mortality rates are falling in men but rising in women
Approximately 220,000 hospital admissions per year
(Mean length of stay 7.5 days)
27 million working days lost per year

Table 4. Epidemiology of COPD in England and Wales.

Pathology and Pathophysiology

Pathology

The pathological changes of COPD are complex and correlate poorly with the physiological abnormalities (Figure 12). There is inflammation in the peripheral airways, fibrosis in airway walls, smooth muscle hypertrophy, goblet cell hyperplasia, mucus hypersecretion and destruction of the lung parenchyma.[56]

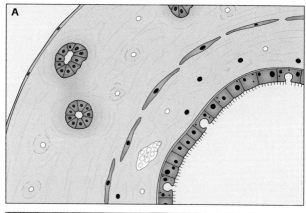

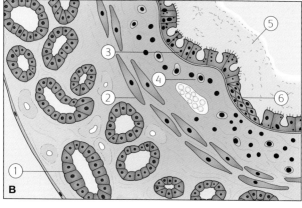

As well as the changes in the airways and lung parenchyma, there are changes in the pulmonary vessels, leading to pulmonary hypertension,[57] and systemic metabolic effects, leading to weight loss.[58] Although characteristic of COPD, some of these changes can be seen in smokers who do not have airflow limitation and they persist even after stopping smoking.[59,60]

Chronic bronchitis (i.e. chronic mucus hypersecretion) is associated with an increase in the volume and number of submucosal glands and the number of goblet cells in the mucosa.

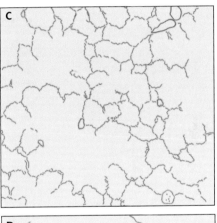

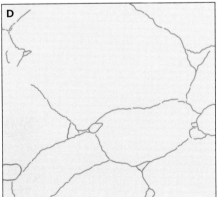

Figure 12. Normal bronchial (A) and lung parenchyma (C) structures and the changes seen in the airways (B) – 1. Mucus gland hypertrophy, 2. Smooth muscle hypertrophy, 3. Goblet cell hyperplasia, 4. Inflammatory cell infiltrate, 5. Excessive mucus, 6. Squamous metaplasia, and (D) parenchyma in COPD.

Emphysema is defined by the pathological changes that occur as "a condition of the lung characterized by abnormal, permanent enlargement of airspaces distal to the terminal bronchiole accompanied by destruction of their walls and without obvious fibrosis". The distribution of the abnormal airspaces allows the classification of emphysema into panacinar, centriacinar and paraseptal (Figure 13).

Panacinar emphysema may be found in the upper or lower lobes, but in α-1 AT deficiency is generally maximal at the base. Centriacinar emphysema is commonest in the upper zones of both upper and lower lobes, and has a closer relationship to cigarette smoking than panacinar disease. The pattern of emphysema has no effect on the clinical symptoms it produces. Bullae are areas of emphysema larger than 1 cm in diameter that are locally overdistended (Figure 14).

Thirty years ago it was shown that the site of airflow obstruction was the small peripheral airways.[61] Pathologically, however, the changes in these airways are subtle, especially when compared to other conditions associated with small airway obstruction, such as bronchiectasis. Bronchioles and small bronchi derive some of their structural integrity from the attachment of surrounding alveolar walls that act like guy ropes to hold open the airway. In the presence of emphysema, some of this support is lost and airflow limitation develops.[62] Other causes of small

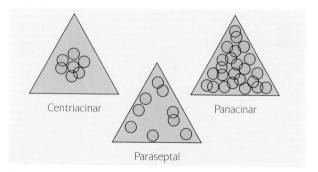

Figure 13. Distribution of the changes found within pulmonary lobules in different types of emphysema.

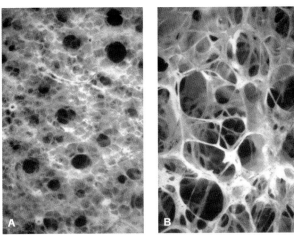

Figure 14. Dissecting microscopic appearance of the cut surface of a normal (A) and emphysematous (B) lung.

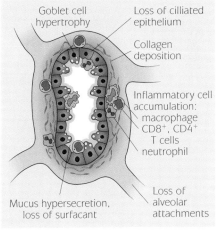

Figure 15.
Mechanisms of small airway narrowing in COPD Reproduced from Shapiro SD. Evolving concepts in the pathogenesis of chronic obstructive pulmonary disease. *Clin Chest Med* 2000; **21**(4): 621–632.[63]

airway obstruction include: increased surface tension as a result of replacement of surfactant by inflammatory exudate; occlusion of the lumen by exudate; oedema and inflammation of the mucosa; and bronchoconstriction (Figure 15).

Cellular mechanisms

Recently, considerable advances have been made in the understanding of the cellular mechanisms involved in the development of COPD. Inflammatory changes are seen in the

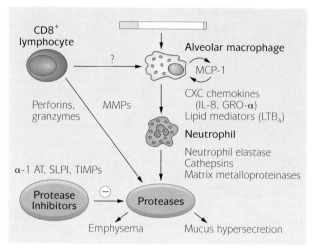

Figure 16. Proposed cellular interactions and inflammatory mediators involved in the airway inflammation seen in COPD. Reproduced with permission from Barnes PJ. Mechanisms in COPD: differences from asthma. *Chest* 2000; **117**(2, Suppl): 10S–4S.[75]

Summary of cellular pathophysiological differences between COPD and Asthma		
	COPD	**Asthma**
Predominant cells in airways	Neutrophils	Eosinophils
Other cells present	Macrophages	CD4+ Th2 lymphocytes
	CD8+ lymphocytes	Mast cells
Principal mediators	LTB4	LTD4
	IL-8	IL-4, IL-5
	TNF-α	

Table 5. Summary of cellular pathophysiological differences between COPD and asthma.

airways of young smokers before structural changes are present.[64] Smoking and COPD are associated with infiltration of the airway wall by CD8[+] T-lymphocytes, and macrophages and neutrophils are found in the airway lumen.[56] The number of CD8[+] cells correlates with the degree of airflow limitation.[65,66] It is thought the neutrophils move rapidly out of capillaries, through the airway wall and into the lumen,[67] and that they are the key inflammatory cells. This is one of the most important differences between asthma and COPD,[68] and it has considerable significance for therapy. Eosinophils are not present in the airway of patients with COPD, but they do appear during exacerbations.[69]

Macrophages may cause damage to the lung through the release of proteinases,[70] and they appear to recruit neutrophils by releasing interleukin-8 (IL-8) and leukotriene B4 (LTB4).[71,72] Macrophages themselves may be activated directly by cigarette smoke or by the CD8[+] T-lymphocytes, which may also damage the lungs directly through the release of tumour necrosis factor alpha (TNFα). Neutrophils release proteolytic enzymes such as neutrophil elastase, cathepsins and matrix metaloproteinases, which may cause the tissue destruction seen in emphysema.[73] The inflammatory activity of neutrophils, lymphocytes and macrophages depends on the production of cAMP, intracellular levels of which are determined by a balance between the activities of protein kinases and phosphodiesterases (Figure 16, Table 5).[74]

Pathophysiology

Decreased maximal expiratory flow and impaired gas exchange are fundamental to the pathophysiology of COPD. The effects of static airway obstruction are exacerbated by the loss of lung recoil due to destruction of the lung parenchyma.

The resting volume of the thorax is determined by the balance between the elastic recoil of the lungs and the chest wall. The floppier the lungs, the less force there is to balance the recoil of the chest wall and thus the resting thoracic volume is increased. This is in part responsible for hyperinflation seen in COPD and the increase in functional residual capacity (FRC) (Figure 17).

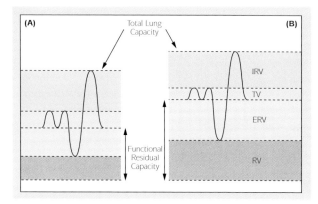

Figure 17. Static lung volumes in a normal subject (A) and a patient with COPD (B).

Loss of lung recoil also means that the airways collapse earlier in expiration (i.e. at larger lung volumes), increasing the amount of air trapped in the lungs and again increasing the FRC and residual volume (RV). Decreased dynamic compliance also leads to the development of hyperinflation. Dynamic hyperinflation develops when the severity of airflow limitation is such that the duration of expiration is insufficient to allow the lungs to deflate fully prior to the next inspiration (Figure 18).

The increase in FRC greatly increases the work of breathing. In COPD, both the force of contraction generated by the inspiratory muscles and the mechanical load against which they are required to act are abnormal.[76] The inspiratory load is increased as a result of the airway obstruction. The force of contraction is reduced as a consequence of: the effect of hyperinflation altering the mechanical advantage of the muscles (both intercostal and diaphragmatic); malnutrition; and, in some cases, respiratory muscle fatigue. Inspiratory muscle dysfunction is central to the development of hypercapnia.[77]

Pulmonary artery hypertension is the most important cardiovascular complication of COPD and it is associated with a poor prognosis.[78] The normal pulmonary circulation is a low-pressure, low-resistance system with low vasomotor tone. The considerable increases seen in cardiac output with exercise do

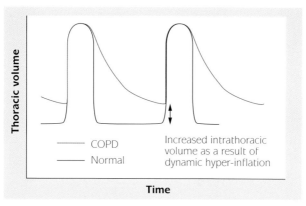

Figure 18. Effect of airflow obstruction and reduced expiratory flow rates on the development of dynamic hyperinflation.

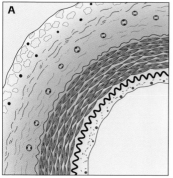

Figure 19. Structure of a normal pulmonary artery (a) and changes seen in pulmonary hypertension (b) – 1.Duplication of elastic laminae and 2.Medial hypertrophy.

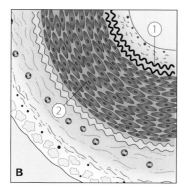

not lead to significant increases in pulmonary artery pressure because they are associated with recruitment of under-perfused vessels, particularly at the lung apex. In hypoxaemic patients with COPD, characteristic changes occur in peripheral pulmonary arteries: the intima of small arteries develops accumulations of smooth muscle; and muscular arteries develop medial hypertrophy (Figure 19).[78] These structural changes may be more important in the development of sustained pulmonary hypertension than hypoxic vasoconstriction.[79] Pulmonary thrombosis may also develop, possibly secondary to small airway inflammation.[80]

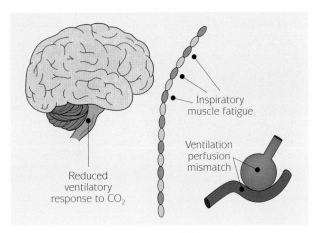

Figure 20. Causes of hypercapnia in COPD.

As described above, some patients with COPD have difficulty in excreting CO_2 as a result of inspiratory muscle fatigue, ventilation perfusion mismatch and possibly alveolar hypoventilation. Some of these patients respond to the difficulty in excreting CO_2 by increasing the frequency and depth of their breathing to maintain a normal arterial partial pressure of CO_2 ($PaCO_2$). However, some patients are unable to maintain adequate alveolar ventilation and there is an adaptive response in the control of breathing, with a reduced ventilatory response to the $PaCO_2$.[81] This leads to a rise in the $PaCO_2$ and the arterial partial pressure of oxygen (PaO_2) becomes an important factor controlling breathing. Some, but not all, of these patients hypoventilate if given too much supplementary oxygen,[82-84] and it is these patients who are at risk of CO_2 narcosis and respiratory arrest. There is a very poor relationship between ventilatory capacity (i.e. FEV_1) and the development of ventilatory failure (Figure 20).[85]

It has recently been recognized that COPD is more than a lung disease and affects other organs, particularly skeletal muscle. The mechanisms of this remain unclear, but probably relate to systemic effects of cytokines, particularly $TNF\alpha$.[58] Loss of muscle mass is an independent predictor of outcome in COPD and is an area infrequently addressed by therapy.[86]

Diagnosis

The key to making a diagnosis of COPD is to think of the diagnosis in smokers who have respiratory symptoms, to confirm the presence of airflow obstruction and to demonstrate that this is largely irreversible.

Many patients will only present at the time of an exacerbation and will be unaware that they have a chronic illness. Some will have had a cough or been breathless for some time, but will not have recognized that these were symptoms of a lung condition. It is often only in retrospect that patients realize that they have been breathless on exertion or have had a productive cough for several years. Many smokers have a morning cough that they regard as normal for them and become breathless on exertion, which they regard as a part of normal ageing. Unless the diagnosis is suspected, specific symptoms sought and the presence of airflow limitation demonstrated, patients will be overlooked.

Most patients have smoked at least 20 cigarettes per day for at least 20 years before they develop symptoms; however, airflow obstruction may develop sooner and is usually present for some years before symptoms develop. If airflow obstruction is detected at this stage, progression to symptomatic COPD may be prevented by stopping the patient smoking. The identification of these pre-symptomatic individuals presents a challenge for health promotion programmes, but now that effective anti-smoking interventions are available there is a greater incentive to try to identify these patients using spirometry as a screening tool.[87]

Smoking cessation is an extremely cost-effective intervention.[88,89] It can be very satisfying for those involved and offers significant cardiovascular benefits, as well as offering the potential to prevent the development of COPD.

Importance of differentiating COPD from asthma

In the past, some of the patients whose symptoms have been identified have been mislabelled as having asthma. They feature on primary care asthma registers and are managed by practice nurses according to asthma protocols. Not surprisingly, they do not respond as well as asthmatics and this frequently leads to unnecessary escalation of treatment, whilst other important management issues are overlooked. Establishing that the correct diagnosis is COPD and not asthma means that patients can be given: a more appropriate prognosis; more realistic expectations of the results of treatment; more appropriate anti-smoking advice; advice on the importance of exercise; and more appropriate and holistic management (Table 6).

History

Patients with mild airflow obstruction are often asymptomatic, but as COPD develops patients become progressively more symptomatic. The relationship of symptoms to different levels of physiological abnormality and the rate of progression can be very variable. Age is a risk factor for COPD, and the presence of symptoms suggestive of a diagnosis of COPD in patients under the age of 40, should raise the possibility of an alternative diagnosis or an unusual aetiology, such as α-1 AT deficiency.

The cardinal symptoms are coughing, wheezing and breathlessness. Patients may present with symptoms occurring on most days, or they may first present at the time of an exacerbation or with an episode of winter bronchitis, or a "chest

Reasons for differentiating COPD from asthma
Different aetiology
Different prognosis
Different therapies
Different response to therapy

Table 6. Reasons for differentiating COPD from asthma.

infection", i.e. a period of increased breathlessness associated with increased production of sputum, which may be purulent. When patients do first develop symptoms, these are usually mild and intermittent. Patients with moderate COPD invariably have some symptoms, but again the spectrum is wide. Patients with severe COPD are almost always breathless on minimal exertion, and their sleep may be disturbed by breathlessness. They generally cough, especially in the mornings, and frequently wheeze. In addition, they may have symptoms of complications such as peripheral oedema.

Coughing

In 75% of patients with COPD, coughing is one of the first symptoms, preceding or developing simultaneously with breathlessness. It may be productive of sputum and is generally worse in the morning. In the absence of infection, the sputum may vary in colour from clear, through white to grey. Purulent (green or brown) sputum can be a sign of infection, but can also simply be a reflection of the neutrophil trafficking seen as part of the inflammatory process.

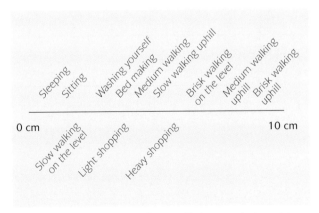

Figure 21. The oxygen cost diagram. Patients mark the point on the line above which they become breathless.

Breathlessness

Breathlessness usually develops insidiously and may be regarded as a normal part of ageing. Patients often modify their behaviour to avoid activities that provoke breathlessness and thus may not experience this symptom.

Subjective breathlessness correlates poorly with the degree of airflow obstruction. It can be quantified by asking about exercise tolerance (for example, the distance the patient can walk on the flat or the number of flights of stairs they can climb before having to stop) or by using a scale such as the oxygen cost diagram (Figure 21) or MRC scale (Table 7).

Unlike asthma, the breathlessness of COPD does not vary markedly from day to day or within a day, and patients' exercise capacity is fairly constant. Breathlessness may vary according to environmental conditions and often worsens in smoky or dusty atmospheres. It is also sensitive to changes in the weather, particularly temperature and humidity. The lack of good and bad days is a useful pointer to the diagnosis of COPD.

MRC dyspnoea scale	
Grade	**Degree of breathlessness related to activities**
0	Not troubled by breathlessness except on strenuous exercise
1	Short of breath when hurrying or walking up a slight hill
2	Walks slower than contemporaries on the level because of breathlessness, or has to stop for breath when walking at own pace
3	Stops for breath after walking about 100 m or after a few minutes on the level
4	Too breathless to leave the house, or breathless when dressing or undressing

Table 7. MRC dyspnoea scale.

Chest pain

Chest pain may be a feature of COPD and is thought to be related to intercostal muscle ischaemia, but other causes such as infection, tumours or ischaemic heart disease should be excluded.

Disability

The disability related to COPD can be assessed by asking about limitations on normal activities such as shopping, gardening, housework, washing, dressing, etc.

Exacerbations

Many patients experience exacerbations and these episodes may be the only symptoms recognized as abnormal by patients. They may present with frequent "chest infections", particularly in the winter. There are often few other symptoms of infection (e.g. fever) and there is often a history of similar episodes.

Patients experience increased breathlessness and have a cough productive of purulent sputum.

Cardiovascular symptoms

Ankle swelling occurs as a consequence of the development of cor pulmonale. It often worsens at times of exacerbations.

Systemic symptoms

Weight loss is a common symptom in advanced COPD. It is due to a combination of the effects of the increased work of breathing, reduced calorie intake because of increased breathlessness and the metabolic effects of COPD. However, it may also be a feature of lung cancer and rapid weight loss, particularly if associated with other symptoms, should always be investigated.

Depression

The exercise limitation, frustration and social isolation produced by COPD often leads to clinical depression (Table 8).

Smoking history

As well as symptoms, it is essential to question patients about their smoking history (Table 9). Current and ex-smokers should be asked at what age they started smoking, the average number of cigarettes smoked per day (or the amount of tobacco per week) and, if they have stopped, when this occurred.

It is conventional to express smoking history in terms of pack years: 20 cigarettes per day for 12 months equals 1 pack year. Smoking 2 oz (50 g) of tobacco per week as self-rolled cigarettes is approximately equivalent to 20 manufactured cigarettes per day. It is more difficult to determine equivalence

Common symptoms
Breathlessness
Cough
Wheeze
Frequent winter "bronchitis"
Depression
Weight loss
Chest pain
Ankle swelling

Table 8. Common symptoms.

Key points in smoking history
Amount of tobacco smoked
Age started smoking
Time to first cigarette in morning
Desire to quit
Passive exposure

Table 9. Key points in smoking history.

Occupational exposures known to cause COPD

Coal mining
Cotton dust
Grain dust
Cement dust
Oil fumes
Cadmium fumes

Table 10. Occupational exposures known to cause COPD.

for pipe tobacco and cigars. Moreover, cigarette yields vary considerably and thus self-reported estimates of tobacco usage are at best an approximation.

Non-smokers should be questioned about passive tobacco smoke exposure both at work and at home.

Other points

The history should also include a detailed occupational history (Table 10), as well as a detailed past medical history including childhood respiratory problems. Many patients are labelled as having COPD when their history reveals other conditions such as bronchiectasis. It is important that these patients are not misdiagnosed as having COPD.

Clinical signs

The findings on clinical examination in patients with COPD are as variable as the symptoms.

Examination is often normal in patients with asymptomatic or mild disease.

In patients with moderate disease there may be signs of hyperinflation (depressed liver, loss of cardiac dullness, reduced crico-sternal distance, increased antero-posterior diameter of

Clinical signs
None
Hyperinflated chest
Wheeze or quiet breath sounds
Purse lip breathing
Use of accessory muscles
Peripheral oedema
Cyanosis
Raised jugular venous pressure (JVP)
Cachexia

Table 11. Clinical signs.

chest). Polyphonic wheezes or abnormally quiet breath sounds may be heard. If there is a component of chronic bronchitis, coarse crackles may be heard. Expiration is prolonged. There is a very poor correlation between the clinical signs and the severity of airflow obstruction.

In patients with severe disease the findings on examination may include: signs of hyperinflation (as above), wheezes, quiet breath sounds, peripheral oedema, elevated venous pressure, central cyanosis, right ventricular heave, loud pulmonary second sound, tricuspid regurgitation, signs of hypercapnia (flapping tremor, bounding pulse, drowsiness), and weight loss or cachexia (Table 11).

Historically, patients have been divided into *blue bloaters* and *pink puffers*. The latter maintain relatively normal blood gases through a drive to breathe that can be extremely distressing. The former are patients who are hypoxaemic and hypercapnic as a result of acclimatization of their regulatory centres and a reduced drive to breathe. They frequently have peripheral oedema as a reflection of pulmonary hypertension and cor pulmonale. In practice these are extremes of a spectrum and most patients lie somewhere in the middle. There is no firm relationship with the predominance of airflow obstruction or emphysema.

Investigations

Investigations are required to confirm the presence of airflow obstruction, to assess whether or not this shows significant variability and to assess the patient for complications, such as polycythaemia, or associated conditions such as lung cancer.

Spirometry

The presence of airflow limitation is best assessed using spirometry. A normal FEV_1 effectively excludes the diagnosis of COPD but a normal peak expiratory flow rate (PEFR) does not. Significant day-to-day or diurnal peak flow variability of more than 20% may suggest a large reversible component to the airflow obstruction, but at low absolute values the spontaneous variability in PEFR may exceed this value.

Spirometry measures the volume of air exhaled in 1 second (the FEV_1) and the total amount of air exhaled (the forced vital capacity, FVC) when the patient inhales maximally and then exhales as forcefully and deeply as possible. By comparing these volumes with those predicted for the patient's age, sex and height, and computing the ratio of the FEV_1 to FVC, it is

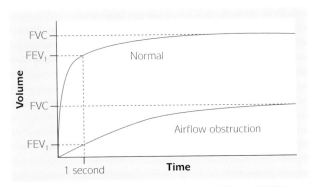

Figure 22. Time–volume curves showing the FEV_1 and FVC in normal subjects and in patients with airflow obstruction due to COPD, for example.

possible to diagnose airflow obstruction with confidence. It is also possible to diagnose mild airflow obstruction and to assess the severity of airflow obstruction (Figure 22).

As well as measuring the FVC, spirometers can be used to measure the vital capacity (VC). This is also known as the slow (or relaxed) vital capacity, as it is measured by asking the patient to exhale fully in a slow, non-forced manner after a maximum inhalation. The VC is often greater then the FVC in diseases such as COPD, where the airways are floppy and collapse prematurely during a forced manoeuvre. In such patients the FEV_1/VC ratio gives a more accurate indication of the degree of airflow obstruction (Table 12).

Spirometry does not itself differentiate between airflow obstruction due to asthma and that due to COPD, but when used in conjunction with reversibility testing it is a sensitive way of diagnosing COPD. Measurement of peak expiratory flow (PEF) rates has proved extremely useful in the monitoring of patients with asthma, but it frequently underestimates the severity of airflow obstruction in COPD. This is because in COPD the airways are generally floppy and the degree of

Example of Use of VC			
	Measured	**Predicted**	**% predicted**
FEV1	0.78 l	2.40 l	33
FVC	1.24 l	2.83 l	44
VC	1.71 l	2.81 l	61
FEV_1/FVC	63%		
FEV_1/VC	46%		

Table 12. Example of use of VC.

Uses of FEV_1 in COPD
Diagnosis (combined with reversibility testing)
Assessing severity
Assessing prognosis
Monitoring progression

Table 13. Uses of FEV_1 in COPD.

airflow obstruction shows significant volume dependency. Thus, at large lung volumes the flow limitation is less severe and the *peak* expiratory flow rate is relatively well preserved, whereas at lower lung volumes the expiratory flow rate is severely limited. This is reflected in a reduction in the FEV_1.

Spirometry has several other advantages over the measurement of PEF rates. It is more reproducible and low readings, due to poor technique or inadequate effort, are easily identified. The British Thoracic Society (BTS) COPD guidelines recommend that spirometry is available in primary care or that an open access service is provided by secondary care. There are many advantages for practices that own their own spirometer, not least the immediacy with which results are available (Table 13).

Types of spirometer Some spirometers measure exhaled volumes directly, but these models are bulky and most spirometers used in primary care measure flow, and integrate electronically over time to derive exhaled volumes. Spirometers should adhere to American Thoracic Society (ATS) standards and need regular calibration, which is quick and easy to do (Table 14). Spirometers also need regular cleaning and servicing.

Making the measurement For the results of spirometry to be meaningful the measurement must be made properly. The BTS with the Association of Respiratory Technicians and Physiologists (ARTP) and the ATS have published guidance on the performance of spirometry.[90,91] Production of reliable results is very dependent on the person performing the test with the

ATS Standards for spirometers	
FEV₁ and FVC Range	0.5 to 8 litres
Accuracy	± 5% reading or ± 0.100 litres, whichever is greater
Reproducibility (precision)	± 3% reading or ± 0.050 litres, whichever is greater
Minimum detectable volume	0.030 litres
Duration of volume acquisition	At least 15 seconds
Display	Paper record or graphical display required

Table 14. ATS standards for spirometers.

patient. They must understand the criteria for an adequate manoeuvre and must have the ability to coax the patient to perform a maximal forced exhalation. They will often need to demonstrate the manoeuvre first. Spirometry is best supervised by people who do it regularly and many practices find it convenient to concentrate the skills in one or two practice nurses.

Patients should be sitting, unless they are very obese. Exhalation should continue for at least 6 seconds and the test should not be stopped until the volume trace has reached a plateau for at least 2 seconds or the exhalation has continued for at least 15 seconds. The results of the measurement should only be accepted if the manoeuvre is performed with maximal effort and if the trace is smooth and cough free (Table 15). The patient should perform at least three manoeuvres and the FVC should be within 5% in two out of the three. The best FEV_1 and the best FVC are recorded.

Common problems are that the previous inspiration was not complete (i.e. total lung capacity was not reached), that exhalation begins before the patient connects to the mouthpiece, that there is a leak between the lips and the mouthpiece, that the exhalation was performed through pursed lips or partially closed teeth, that the exhalation was not

Criteria for an acceptable spirometric manoeuvre

Full inspiration
Good seal with mouthpiece
Maximum effort used
No coughing
No premature inhalation
Exhalation continues for at least 6 seconds
Volume trace has reached a plateau

Table 15. Criteria for an acceptable spirometric manoeuvre.

Common problems when performing spirometry

Incomplete inhalation
Exhalation begun before connected to mouthpiece
Air leak around mouthpiece
Exhalation through pursed lips
Exhalation not maximally forced
Exhalation not complete
Coughing during exhalation

Table 16. Common problems when performing spirometry.

maximally forced or sustained to residual volume, and that the exhalation was interrupted by coughing or premature inhalation (Table 16).

Interpreting the results of spirometry The results of spirometry must be interpreted in the light of the predicted values for that patient. The reference values most commonly used in Europe are those produced by a working party of the European Respiratory Society (Tables 17 and 18).[92] Many spirometers now calculate the predicted values for an individual once their age, sex and height have been entered, but tables of normal values are widely available.

Predicted values for FEV$_1$ and FVC in men (From ref (92))							
Age		Height					
		5' 3" 160cm	5' 5" 165cm	5' 7" 170cm	5' 9" 175cm	5' 11" 180cm	6' 1" 185cm	6' 3" 190cm
38-41	FEV$_1$	3.20	3.42	3.63	3.85	4.06	4.28	4.49
	FVC	3.81	4.10	4.39	4.67	4.96	5.25	5.54
42-45	FEV$_1$	3.09	3.30	3.52	3.73	3.95	4.16	4.38
	FVC	3.71	3.99	4.28	4.57	4.86	5.15	5.43
46-49	FEV$_1$	2.97	3.18	3.40	3.61	3.83	4.04	4.26
	FVC	3.60	3.89	4.18	4.47	4.75	5.04	5.33
50-53	FEV$_1$	2.85	3.07	3.28	3.50	3.71	3.93	4.14
	FVC	3.50	3.79	4.07	4.36	4.65	4.94	5.23
54-57	FEV$_1$	2.74	2.95	3.17	3.38	3.60	3.81	4.03
	FVC	3.39	3.68	3.97	4.26	4.55	4.83	5.12
58-61	FEV$_1$	2.62	2.84	3.05	3.27	3.48	3.70	3.91
	FVC	3.29	3.58	3.87	4.15	4.44	4.73	5.02
62-65	FEV$_1$	2.51	2.72	2.94	3.15	3.37	3.58	3.80
	FVC	3.19	3.47	3.76	4.05	4.34	4.63	4.91
66-69	FEV$_1$	2.39	2.60	2.82	3.03	3.25	3.46	3.68
	FVC	3.08	3.37	3.66	3.95	4.23	4.52	4.81

Table 17. Predicted values for FEV$_1$ and FVC in men (from Ref. 92).

Reversibility testing Spirometry alone cannot diagnose COPD; it will merely show the presence of airflow obstruction. Reversibility testing is central to making the diagnosis of fixed or substantially irreversible airflow limitation. In practice there is a spectrum of reversibility that overlaps with asthma. Reversibility can be assessed acutely with short-acting bronchodilators or over a period of weeks with oral or inhaled corticosteroids.

Reversibility testing with bronchodilators should be carried out in a way that ensures that a failure to respond is not because the dose is too low. For this reason it is best to use nebulized drugs, and both beta agonists (such as salbutamol or terbutaline)

Age		4' 11" 150cm	5' 1" 155cm	5' 3" 160cm	5' 5" 165cm	5' 7" 170cm	5' 9" 175cm	5' 11" 180cm
					Height			
38-41	FEV_1	2.30	2.50	2.70	2.89	3.09	3.29	3.49
	FVC	2.69	2.91	3.13	3.35	3.58	3.8	4.02
42-45	FEV_1	2.20	2.40	2.60	2.79	2.99	3.19	3.39
	FVC	2.59	2.81	3.03	3.25	3.47	3.69	3.91
46-49	FEV_1	2.10	2.30	2.50	2.69	2.89	3.09	3.29
	FVC	2.48	2.70	2.92	3.15	3.37	3.59	3.81
50-53	FEV_1	2.00	2.20	2.40	2.59	2.79	2.99	3.19
	FVC	2.38	2.60	2.82	3.04	3.26	3.48	3.71
54-57	FEV_1	1.90	2.10	2.30	2.49	2.69	2.89	3.09
	FVC	2.27	2.49	2.72	2.94	3.16	3.38	3.60
58-61	FEV_1	1.80	2.00	2.20	2.39	2.49	2.69	2.89
	FVC	2.17	2.39	2.61	2.83	3.06	3.28	3.50
62-65	FEV_1	1.70	1.90	2.10	2.29	2.49	2.69	2.89
	FVC	2.07	2.29	2.51	2.73	2.95	3.17	3.39
66-69	FEV_1	1.60	1.80	2.00	2.19	2.39	2.59	2.79
	FVC	1.96	2.18	2.40	2.63	2.85	3.07	3.29

Predicted values for FEV_1 and FVC in women (From ref (92))

Table 18. Predicted values for FEV_1 and FVC in women (from Ref. 92).

and anticholinergics should be used either sequentially or in combination. For simplicity and to maximize the predictive value of the test, it is best to use a combination of salbutamol and ipratropium delivered via a nebulizer (Table 19).

Tests should be performed when patients are clinically stable and free of infection. The patient should not have taken a short-acting bronchodilator in the previous 6 hours, a long-acting beta agonist in the previous 12 hours or a sustained release theophylline preparation in the previous 24 hours.

The response should be assessed by measuring the pre- and post-trial FEV_1. An increase in FEV_1 that is both more than 200 ml and more than 15% of the pre-test value is the

Bronchodilator reversibility testing protocol

Patient must be clinically stable
Patients should avoid:
    short-acting beta agonist for 6 hours
    long-acting beta agonist for 12 hours
    sustained release theophylline for 24 hours.
Baseline spirometry
Nebulize salbutamol (2.5 mg) and ipratropium (500 mg)
Wait 30 minutes
Repeat spirometry

Table 19. Bronchodilator reversibility testing protocol.

Interpretation of reversibility test results

A positive reversibility is one when the increase
in post-bronchodilator FEV_1 is both:
    greater than 200 ml
    and
    shows a 15% increase over the pre-bronchodilator value

Table 20. Interpretation of reversibility test results.

threshold recommended by the BTS for establishing reversibility (Table 20).

The post-test FEV_1 also gives information about prognosis, but the acute response to bronchodilators in this setting has relatively little bearing on the subsequent subjective or objective response to bronchodilator therapy: a negative result does not mean that patients will not derive symptomatic benefits, in terms of perception of breathlessness and increases in walking distance, from treatment with bronchodilators.

Steroid reversibility testing is not usually required in patients with mild disease, but should be carried out in all patients with moderate and severe disease. FEV_1 should be measured before and at the end of a course of oral steroids. A positive response will usually be produced in patients treated with 30 mg prednisolone daily within 2 weeks, but some clinicians continue the trial for up to 4 weeks. Inhaled steroids can also be used, but in this case the trial should continue for 6 weeks with doses equivalent to 1000 µg beclomethasone per day, and a negative response may be influenced by poor compliance or inhaler technique.

The criteria for a positive response are the same as for trials of bronchodilators, and a rise in FEV_1 of more than 200 ml is associated with a better prognosis over the next 5 years.

Some patients report a subjective improvement following steroid therapy, but do not show a significant increase in their FEV_1. Such patients should not be considered as having a positive response and should not continue on oral corticosteroids. Failure to respond to a steroid trial when clinically stable does not mean that patients should not receive steroids during an exacerbation because different inflammatory cells are involved at these times (Table 21).

Assessing the severity of COPD using spirometry The BTS guidelines propose a classification of COPD into mild, moderate and severe based on FEV_1. Patients' health needs are related to these categories and exacerbation rates, and the risk of hospitalization increase as the FEV_1 falls.

Steroid reversibility testing protocols

Spirometry before and after:
2 weeks treatment with 30 mg prednisolone daily.
6 weeks treatment with 800 mcg to1,000 mcg inhaled steroids daily.

Table 21. Steroid reversibility testing protocols.

Guidelines on the management of COPD, containing recommendations on severity assessment, have also been published by the American Thoracic Society, the European Respiratory Society (ERS) and most recently by the Global Initiative for Chronic Obstructive Lung Disease (GOLD).[8,9,93] All four define severity in slightly different ways. The BTS, ERS and GOLD guidelines use definitions based on both the FEV_1/FVC ratio and the FEV_1. The BTS and GOLD guidelines recommend that the absolute value of the ratio should be less than 70%, whereas the ERS recommends that the FEV_1/FVC ratio must be less than 88% predicted. All three use the FEV_1 (as a percentage of the predicted) to define severity (Table 22).

In COPD, the post-bronchodilator FEV_1 is a useful predictor of mortality, but it relates poorly to health status (Figure 23).

Recommendations for severity grading in COPD using spirometry			
Severity	BTS	ERS	GOLD
At Risk	Not defined	Not defined	Normal spirometry Cough & Sputum
Mild	FEV_1 60–80%	FEV_1/FVC <88% predicted and FEV_1 ≥70%	FEV_1/FVC <70% and FEV_1 >80%
Moderate	FEV_1 40–60%	FEV_1/FVC <88% predicted and FEV_1 50–69%	FEV_1/FVC <70% and FEV_1 <80% and ≥ 30%
Severe	FEV_1 <40%	FEV_1/FVC <88% predicted and FEV_1 ≤50%	FEV_1/FVC <70% and FEV_1 <30% Or FEV_1 <50% and signs of respiratory or right heart failure

Table 22. Recommendations for severity grading in COPD using spirometry.

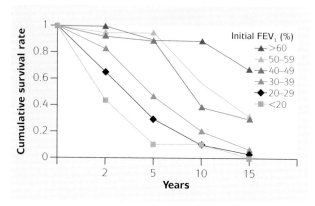

Figure 23. Relationship between FEV_1 as a percentage of predicted end mortality. Reproduced with permission from Traver GA *et al.* Predictors of mortality in chronic obstructive pulmonary disease. A 15-year follow-up study. *Am Rev Respir Dis* 1979; **119**(6): 895–902.[94]

Training in spirometry Training in the use of spirometers and interpretation of the results is widely available. Many hospitals offer training in spirometry for their local primary care teams. Spirometry training is also provided nationally by organizations such as the National Respiratory Training Centre (NRTC) or the Respiratory Education Resource Centres. For those wanting a more academic qualification, the BTS/ARTP offer a certificate in spirometry. Candidates are required to achieve a satisfactory standard in a practical examination, an oral examination and an assignment. Many manufacturers also offer instruction and advice on the correct use of their spirometers.

Detailed lung function testing

Laboratory lung function tests measuring static lung volumes [total lung capacity (TLC), residual volume (RV) and functional residual capacity (FRC) (see Figure 17)] and gas transfer are useful in some patients, particularly those in whom the level of

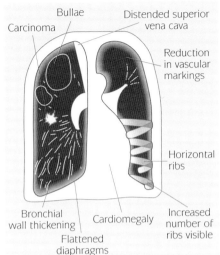

Figure 24. Diagram showing abnormalities that may be seen on the plain chest radiograph in patients with COPD.

Labels in figure:
- Carcinoma
- Bullae
- Distended superior vena cava
- Reduction in vascular markings
- Horizontal ribs
- Increased number of ribs visible
- Cardiomegaly
- Flattened diaphragms
- Bronchial wall thickening

breathlessness or functional impairment appears disproportionate to the degree of airflow limitation measured by spirometry.

Radiology

The plain chest radiograph is frequently unremarkable in patients with stable mild disease. As such, it contributes little to the diagnosis but its role lies in excluding other diagnoses such as a bronchogenic carcinoma. It may show hyperinflation, bronchial wall thickening, a paucity of vascular markings or single or multiple bullae, but may be surprisingly normal in patients with significant emphysema as assessed by gas transfer measurements or by CT.

In patients with exacerbations, plain chest radiographs are again principally useful for excluding other causes of the patient's symptoms, such as lobar pneumonia or pneumothorax (Figure 24). Follow-up films are only indicated if there is a serious deterioration in the patient's existing symptoms or if new symptoms develop.

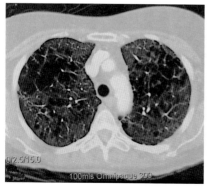

Figure 25.
Appearances of emphysema on high-resolution CT.

CT is good at showing the presence of emphysema, but is only rarely clinically indicated for this purpose (Figure 25). Examples of its use are as part of a work up for bullectomy, lung volume reduction surgery or single lung transplantation, and to confirm the presence of emphysema in young patients with isolated low gas transfer measurements (e.g. α-1 AT deficiency).

Pulse oximetry and arterial blood gas tensions

Pulse oximetry can be used to assess hypoxaemia at rest and on exertion in patients with stable disease and during exacerbations. If the SaO_2 is more than 92% in patients with stable disease, measurement of arterial blood gas tensions is probably not required. If the SaO_2 is < 92%, arterial blood gas tensions should be measured and measurement of arterial blood gases should be considered in all patients with an exacerbation as their $PaCO_2$ may be abnormal even if their SaO_2 is normal.

Sleep studies

Some patients with COPD are not hypoxic during the day but desaturate at night (SaO_2 < 90% for more than 30% of the night). These patients do not appear to gain any survival advantage from nocturnal oxygen therapy and treatment does not delay the need for long-term oxygen therapy (see p. 81).[95–97]

Unless patients with COPD have unexplained cor pulmonale or polycythaemia or have symptoms of co-existing obstructive sleep apnoea, overnight sleep studies are not necessary.

Electro- and echocardiography

The ECG is useful for detecting ischaemic heart disease and arrhythmias, but is relatively insensitive for detecting right ventricular hypertrophy. ECG criteria for ventricular hypertrophy are modified by hyperinflation of the lungs.

Echocardiography is a useful way of identifying right ventricular hypertrophy and dilatation; however, hyperinflation increases the retrosternal air space, thus making satisfactory transthoracic studies difficult. Where available, transoesophageal echocardiography increases the proportion of satisfactory examinations. Pulmonary artery (PA) pressure, can be estimated using echocardiography in a number of ways. The blood velocity in the main PA can be used to estimate the PA pressure, and the interval between the onset of RV ejection and peak velocity correlates well with the mean PA pressure. In patients with tricuspid regurgitation, the addition of the mean right atrial (RA) pressure to the peak systolic gradient between the RA and RV yields the systolic pulmonary artery pressure.

Haematology

Identification of anaemia and polycythaemia is useful in the management of patients with COPD. Patients with a haematocrit >47% in women or >52% in men should be investigated for hypoxaemia, including at night. Venesection should be considered if the PCV is greater than 60% in men or 55% in women; however, the evidence for its benefits in terms of improved exercise performance and reduced risk of vascular events is limited, as is evidence regarding the duration of benefit.

Sputum culture

Routine sputum culture is of no value in the management of patients with stable COPD. Sputum is frequently colonized with bacteria such as *Haemophilus influenzae*, whose identification, in itself, is not an indication for antibiotic therapy.

Summary of other available investigations

Full blood count
Chest radiograph
ECG
Sputum culture
Pulse oximetry
Arterial blood gases
Detailed lung function testing
Echocardiogram
Sleep study

Table 23. Summary of other available investigations.

During an acute exacerbation, sputum usually becomes purulent and this is one of the defining features. A Gram stain may show a mixture of organisms, similar to those cultures when the patient is stable. These may include *Streptococcus pneumoniae*, *Haemophilus influenzae* and *Moraxella catarrhalis*. If thought appropriate, antibiotic therapy is usually started before the results of sputum culture are available, but occasionally has to be modified on the basis of culture results and lack of response to empirical therapy (see Table 23 for a summary of the different investigations available).

Differentiation of COPD from asthma

In most cases, the history, examination and investigations will enable patients with asthma to be distinguished from those with COPD (Table 24). Particular pointers are the age of the patient, their smoking history and evidence of variability in airflow obstruction (either serial PEF or reversibility testing). This distinction is important (see p. 33) and attempts should be made to accurately classify all patients.

Differential diagnosis of COPD

The differential diagnosis of patients presenting with symptoms suggestive of COPD is shown in Table 25. The differentiation

Pointers that differentiate asthma from COPD

	COPD	Asthma
History		
Smoker or ex-smoker	Nearly all	Possibly
Symptoms under age 45	Uncommon	Often
Chronic *productive* cough	Common	Uncommon
Breathlessness	Persistent and progressive	Variable
Winter bronchitis	Common	Uncommon
Investigations		
Serial PEF	Obstructive picture	May be normal Day to day and diurnal variation
Reversibility testing	Minimal variation Usually <15% or 200 ml change	Usually >15% or 200 ml change

Table 24. Pointers that differentiate asthma from COPD.

Differential diagnosis of COPD

Asthma
Bronchiectasis
Left ventricular dysfunction
Carcinoma of the bronchus
Obliterative bronchiolitis

Table 25. Differential diagnosis of COPD.

of asthma from COPD has been discussed above. Some patients will have both COPD and left ventricular dysfunction, but in others the symptoms will be entirely due to another condition (e.g. bronchiectasis) and these patients may require referral for a specialist opinion.

Prevention

Smoking cessation

Stopping patients smoking is the single most effective way of altering the outcome in patients at all stages in COPD. This is as true for presymptomatic patients with airflow obstruction as it is for patients with severe disease. Those who continue to smoke will continue to lose FEV_1 at an accelerated rate, and although lost function cannot be regained, those who stop smoking will deteriorate more slowly and derive more benefit from therapies such as oxygen (Figure 26).

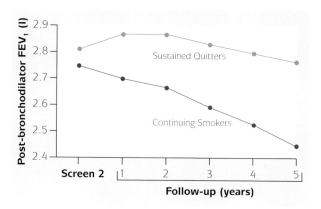

Figure 26. Mean FEV_1 in sustained quitters and continuing smokers in the Lung Health Study. Reproduced with permission from Anthonisen NR *et al*. Effects of smoking intervention and the use of an inhaled anticholinergic bronchodilator on the rate of decline of FEV_1. The Lung Health Study. *J Am Med Assoc* 1994; **272**(19): 1497–1505.[98]

Advice about stopping smoking should be given at every opportunity. Successful quitters consistently list advice from a health professional as one of the main motivational factors for stopping smoking and even brief advice can significantly improve quit rates.

Pharmacotherapy using nicotine replacement improves quit rates and bupropion, particularly when used in conjunction with psychological support, can result in sustained cessation for 12 months in around 25% of smokers. In patients with COPD, sustained cessation rates at 6 months are around 16%.[99]

Familial α-1 AT deficiency

There are conflicting views about whether the relatives of a patient with α-1 AT deficiency should be screened for α-1 AT deficiency themselves.[100] If they are to be screened it is recommended that relatives should be informed of the possibility of a genetic abnormality by the family member who is the index case, rather than by a direct approach from a doctor.[101] The main point of identifying asymptomatic family members is to ensure that they do not smoke, as replacement therapy is of unproven benefit.

Occupation

Workers in dusty occupations associated with the development of COPD should be strongly advised not to smoke, and they should be provided with, and wear, appropriate and effective respiratory protection in the workplace.

Treatment

The treatment of COPD includes drug therapy, surgery, exercise and counselling/psychological support. When managing COPD patients, it is particularly important to evaluate the social and family circumstances, and not to treat the patient in isolation. Interventions at home, such as the installation of a stair lift, may have a considerably greater impact on a patient's quality of life than adding another drug therapy.

Management of symptomatic patients centres around the relief of symptoms, optimization of lung function, improvement in activities, prevention of exacerbations and prevention of complications. The holy grail of COPD management is to prevent or reduce disease progression, but at present the only treatment known to achieve this is long-term oxygen therapy in chronically hypoxic patients.

Guidelines

Guidelines on the management of COPD were published by the BTS in 1997.[2] North American guidelines on the management of COPD[7] and a European Consensus Statement[8] were published in 1995. These are all under revision, but the latest COPD guidelines come from the Global Initiative for Chronic Obstructive Lung Disease (GOLD).[9] This initiative was established by the US National Heart, Lung & Blood Institute (NHLBI) in conjunction with the World Health Organization (WHO). Its goals are "to increase awareness of COPD and decrease mortality and morbidity" from COPD by encouraging research and making consensus-based recommendations on management of COPD.

Assessing the outcome of interventions

Traditionally, the effects of interventions have been assessed by measuring changes in the FEV_1 but, by definition, there is

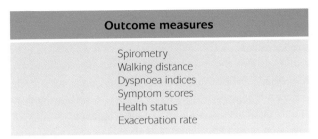

Outcome measures
Spirometry
Walking distance
Dyspnoea indices
Symptom scores
Health status
Exacerbation rate

Table 26. Outcome measures.

limited scope for this to change and other outcome measures must be considered (Table 26). Other spirometric indices such as the slow vital capacity (SVC) and inspiratory capacity (IC) may correlate better with the clinical response to therapy;[102] improvements in patient-centred outcomes such as symptoms, exercise capacity and health status may occur without significant changes in FEV_1[103] and reductions in the frequency of exacerbations may also be relevant. Studies showing differences in these alternative outcome measures must be sufficiently powered to allow interpretation.

Smoking cessation

Smoking cessation advice and therapy remain crucial in all patients with COPD, whatever the severity.[104,105] Stopping smoking returns the accelerated rate of decline in FEV_1 seen in smokers (Figure 4) back to the normal rate.[12,106] Basic anti-smoking advice should be given to all smokers as part of an integrated service offering counselling and support.[107] Recent advances in the pharmacotherapy of nicotine addiction have led to significantly higher quit rates[108] and bupropion has been shown to be effective in patients with COPD.[99] Demonstrating to patients that their lungs have already been damaged by smoking by performing spirometry also appears to improve quit rates.[109]

Drug therapy in stable disease

Bronchodilators

Although the disease is characterized by substantially irreversible airflow obstruction, bronchodilators are still the mainstay of pharmacotherapy.[2,9] Beta agonists, anticholinergics and theophylline are all effective bronchodilators in COPD. The choice of therapy depends on individual responses.

The structural changes in the airways prevent bronchodilators returning airway calibre to normal, and clinically relevant improvements in FEV_1 may be too small to identify against the background day-to-day variation. Inhaled agents are preferred to oral because of the reduction in systemic side-effects. Beta agonists act directly on bronchial smooth muscle to cause bronchodilation, whereas anticholinergics act by inhibiting resting broncho-motor tone. Both classes of drugs act synergistically to reduce airway resistance and reduce hyperinflation (Figure 27).

As discussed above, single dose bronchodilator reversibility tests are important in the assessment of patients with COPD;

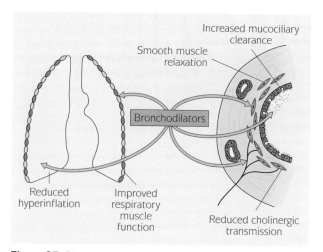

Figure 27. Diagram showing the effects of bronchodilators on airways and respiratory mechanics in patients with COPD.

however, they do not predict the symptomatic benefit that patients may obtain from bronchodilator therapy.[110] Bronchodilators may increase FEV_1, FVC or exercise tolerance independently, but an increase in FEV_1 does not correlate well with an improvement in symptoms. As well as increasing airway calibre, these drugs lead to a reduction in pulmonary hyperinflation, increase mucociliary clearance and improve respiratory muscle function.[111] All of these actions may contribute to the clinical benefit, but most trials have only used changes in FEV_1 as the outcome measure.

Short-acting beta agonists Beta agonists are the most widely used bronchodilators for COPD. The dose–response relationship for salbutamol in patients with largely or completely irreversible COPD is almost flat.[112,113] The time to peak response is slower than in asthmatics and the side-effect to benefits ratio is such that there is little benefit in giving more than 1 mg salbutamol. They are effective for up to 4 hours and can be used both on a regular or an as required basis.

Patients who do not have a significant spirometric response may still benefit if alternative outcome measures such as walking distances are assessed. Studies comparing short-acting beta agonist with placebo have shown significant increases in FEV_1, PEF and symptom scores (Table 27).[114] Beta agonists do not have any significant effect on cough or sputum production, and their effects on walking distance have been inconsistent.

Long-acting beta agonists The physiological effects of long-acting beta agonists are similar to the short-acting agents, but

Effects of short-acting beta agonists

Increased FEV_1
Reduced breathlessness
Increased exercise capacity
Improved health status

Table 27. Effects of short-acting beta agonists.

their duration of action is around 12 hours. Salmeterol has a slower onset of action than eformoterol.

Some patients with COPD undoubtedly get symptomatic benefit. Studies have shown that they produce improvements of approximately 100–200 ml in FEV_1 and they improve health status and breathlessness scores (Table 28).[115–119] These effects are dose dependent and maximum improvement in health status is produced by salmeterol (50 μg) or eformoterol (12 μg) twice daily.[118,119] Larger doses have a reduced effect.

Long-acting beta agonists appear to reduce exacerbation rates in COPD, but the mechanism responsible for this remains unclear. Effects on host defences have been proposed,[120] but it is possible that the effects are due to a reduction in baseline breathlessness, which leads to reduced recognition of exacerbations as a result of increased tolerance of the increased breathlessness that occurs.

Long-acting beta agonists are more expensive than short-acting drugs, but in patients who respond they are more convenient.

Anticholinergics Cholinergic nerves are the main neural bronchoconstrictor pathway in the airways and the resting tone is increased in patients with COPD.[121] Cholinergic effects on the airway are mediated by muscarinic receptors and these also mediate effects on mucus secretion. Three muscarinic receptors are now recognized: M_1 receptors mediate cholinergic transmission in parasympathetic ganglia, M_2 receptors mediate feedback inhibition of acetylcholine (ACh) release from

Effects of long-acting beta agonists
Improved FEV_1
Reduced symptoms
Increased exercise tolerance
Improved health status
Reduced exacerbation rate

Table 28. Effects of long-acting beta agonists.

preganglionic nerves and M3 receptors mediate smooth muscle contraction (Figure 28). Effective anticholinergic drugs block M_1 and M_3 receptors in preference to M_2 receptors, as inhibition of these facilitates ACh release.[122]

The speed of onset of action of ipratropium and oxitropium is slower than short-acting beta agonists, but they produce more sustained bronchodilatation (up to 8 hours) and are at least as effective, and possibly more so.[124–126] Unlike the beta agonists, anticholinergic bronchodilators have also been shown to have a beneficial effect on sleep quality in patients with COPD.[127] The optimal dose of ipratropium is around 80 µg, which is higher that the dose usually prescribed.[128]

A long-acting anticholinergic bronchodilator (tiotropium bromide) which can be given once daily[129] and which has kinetic

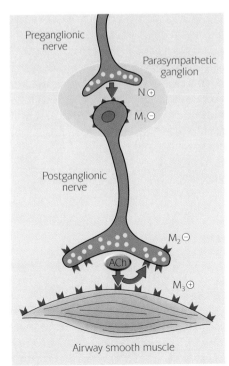

Figure 28. The roles of muscarinic cholinergic receptors in the airways. Reproduced with permission from Barnes PJ. Modulation of neuro-transmission in airways. *Physiol Rev* 1992; **72**(3): 699–729.[123]

selectivity for M_1 and M_3 receptors[130] has recently been developed. This appears to be an effective bronchodilator which reduces breathlessness, improves exercise tolerance, reduces exacerbations and improves health status.[129,131,132]

Anticholinergic bronchodilators should be tried in patients who remain symptomatic despite using short-acting beta agonists. They may be used as combination therapy (see below) or alone, but current guidelines suggest that combination therapy is best reserved for patients who fail to get adequate symptom relief from single agent therapy (Table 29).

Combination therapy Giving short-acting beta agonists at the same time as anticholinergic bronchodilators leads to greater increases in FEV_1, or other measures of airway calibre, than either alone.[133–136] Combination therapy may produce greater symptom relief with fewer side-effects than increasing the dose of a single agent, but may be more expensive. Inhalers containing combinations of ipratropium and salbutamol are also available and offer greater convenience.[126]

Methylxanthines The mechanism of action of methylxanthines remains uncertain.[137] Their primary effect is generally assumed to be relaxation of airway smooth muscle; however, at therapeutic concentrations they have little direct bronchodilator effect. Theophyllines are used in COPD but their use is declining.[138]

Sustained release, oral theophylline and aminophyline produce symptomatic relief and improvements in FEV_1.[139,140]

Effects of anticholinergics
Improved FEV_1
Reduced symptoms
Increased exercise tolerance
Reduced exacerbations
Improved health status
Improved sleep quality

Table 29. Effects of anticholinergics.

They appear to be less effective than long-acting beta agonists[141] and as such are now usually reserved as third-line therapy, usually in combination with inhaled therapy.[142]

Because of potential toxicity and significant interactions with other drugs,[143] they require monitoring of plasma concentrations.[144] The therapeutic index of theophylline is narrow and some patients experience significant side-effects, even when the plasma levels are in the therapeutic range. Ageing-associated changes in liver function lead to a greater risk of toxicity in the elderly.[145] For most patients a measurement of plasma theophylline concentrations 8–10 hours following a single oral dose will be sufficient to predict maintenance requirements and a repeat measurement 1–2 weeks later will confirm that the plasma concentration is in the therapeutic range. Thereafter, monitoring is not necessary unless there has be a change in concomitant medication or the patient's condition that would lead to altered theophylline clearance (Table 30).

Corticosteroids

Although inflammatory changes are present in the airways of patients with COPD, the role of corticosteroids remains controversial.

Oral steroids At best, trials of oral corticosteroids in patients with stable disease have shown improvements in small subsets (15–40%);[146] however, this may be achieved at considerable cost in terms of side-effects and at present there is no means

Theophylline
Used third-line when fail to respond to inhaled beta agonists and anticholinergics
Side-effects (nausea and tachycardia) may be problematic
Plasma concentrations need monitoring
Plasma levels affected by concomitant therapy and smoking

Table 30. Theophylline.

of predicting those who will respond. Less than half of those patients who show objective improvements with oral therapy maintain the improvement on inhaled corticosteroid therapy.[147]

Trials of oral steroid therapy can help to identify patients with significant untreated chronic asthmatic component to their disease,[148] who may benefit from being managed according to asthma protocols, but they are poor predictors of response to inhaled steroids in patients with COPD.[149] Nevertheless, current guidelines recommend that patients showing a good response to oral corticosteroids should be treated along similar lines to asthmatics.[2]

Uncontrolled retrospective studies have suggested that oral corticosteroid therapy can slow the decline in FEV_1, but there is insufficient evidence to recommend this.

The role of oral steroids (Table 31) in the management of acute exacerbations is discussed later (p. 74).

Oral steroids carry with them a dose- and duration-dependent risk of systemic side-effects.[150] There is some individual variability in the susceptibility to the development of side-effects. Patients may notice increased appetite, fluid retention and mood swings with short-term treatment. With longer term, high dose treatment patients may develop skin thinning, easy bruising, weight gain, osteoporosis, cataracts, proximal myopathy, diabetes and hypertension. Patients should be made aware of these effects and when appropriate they should be prescribed therapy (such as hormone or bisphosphonate therapy) to reduce the risk of osteoporosis.

Role of oral steroids

Identification of patients with significant asthmatic component
Speed recovery from an exacerbation
Delay time to next exacerbation
Produce sustained reduction in symptoms in a very small proportion of patients
Significant risk of side-effects

Table 31. Role of oral steroids.

Inhaled steroids The role of inhaled steroids in stable COPD is controversial and has been the subject of four recent large trials.[151–154] All used changes in the rate of decline in FEV_1 as the primary end-point and showed no benefit. Inhaled steroids appear to reduce the number of exacerbations in patients with severe COPD[153–155] and this may be the main benefit of treatment (Table 32). High dose inhaled steroids in patients with COPD may reduce bone mineral density[154] and the benefits must be balanced against such side-effects.[150] Inhaled steroids should be reserved for patients with severe COPD (FEV_1 <40% predicted) who are having frequent exacerbations.

Delivery systems

As with asthma, delivery of the drugs to the lungs is an essential part of pharmacotherapy. When considering delivery devices, co-existing problems, such as arthritis, must be taken into account. Pressurized metered dose inhalers (pMDIs) are cheap but unless used with large-volume spacers give poor pulmonary deposition, and as many as three-quarters of patients with COPD are unable to use them correctly.[156] Dry powder devices are more expensive but can be used successfully by up to 90% of patients and thus may be significantly more cost-effective. Many elderly patients soon forget how to use their inhalers correctly[157] and it is essential to check their inhaler technique at every opportunity and re-instruct as necessary.

Role of inhaled steroids
No effect on disease progression
May reduce exacerbation rates in patients with severe disease
May slow rate of decline in health status

Table 32. Role of inhaled steroids.

Large-volume spacers The use of large-volume spacers with metered dose inhalers is a well-established method of maximizing pulmonary drug deposition in patients with asthma, but there have been few studies in COPD. Poor co-ordination may significantly impair an elderly patient's ability to use a metered dose inhaler and this can be improved using a large-volume spacer (see Table 33).[156]

Nebulizers Most patients achieve maximum possible bronchodilatation with drugs administered by conventional inhalers, but a few derive benefit from very high doses of bronchodilators.[158,159] These high doses are most conveniently delivered using a nebulizer. Some patients may also derive benefits from the moistening or cooling effects of the aerosol generated by a nebulizer, but there is conflicting evidence about whether there is any advantage in delivering the same doses of drugs delivered by inhaler or nebulizer.[160–164]

Compressors to drive nebulizers are relatively cheap, but the drug costs are high and patients may experience more severe systemic effects. For a few patients, there does appear to be a

---

Factors affecting choice of delivery systems

Dexterity
Hand grip strength
Co-ordination
Severity of airflow limitation

Table 33. Factors affecting choice of delivery systems.

Indications for nebulized therapy

Persistent symptoms despite adequate
  bronchodilators therapy from inhalers
Inability to use inhalers
Exacerbations

Table 34. Indications for nebulized therapy.

small advantage in using nebulized therapy, but these patients should have tried maximal doses of inhaled therapy, have had a trial of oral steroids and have a formal assessment of the efficacy of nebulized therapy.[165]

The BTS nebulizer guidelines make recommendations about the assessment of patients for nebulizer therapy.[165] As discussed earlier, patients may derive significant symptomatic benefit from nebulized therapy compared with inhaled therapy without having a significant change in FEV_1. This limits the value of objective assessments of nebulizer therapy and the best assessment may simply be to ask the patients whether they are able to do more, or whether they have fewer symptoms as a result of using nebulized bronchodilators and whether or not they have experienced any adverse effects.

The role of nebulized therapy during exacerbations is discussed on p. 73. They are frequently used despite the fact that there is again conflicting evidence about the comparative efficacy of the same doses of drug given by nebulizer and inhaler. Nebulizers are often preferred because they are easier to administer[166] and because drug deposition is not dependent on inspiratory effort (Table 34).

Indications for referral for a specialist opinion

Most patients with COPD can be managed in primary care but some may require referral to a specialist (Table 35). This may

Indications for referral
Diagnostic uncertainty
Disproportionate symptoms
Persistent symptoms
Development of lung cancer
Pulmonary rehabilitation
Nebulizer assessment
Oxygen assessment

Table 35. Indications for referral.

be because of diagnostic uncertainty (see p. 33), the presence of symptoms that seem out of proportion to the measured lung function abnormality, or for advice on management of persistent symptoms. Patients who have symptoms suggestive of the development of lung cancer (e.g. haemoptysis or weight loss) should be referred urgently. Patients may need to be referred for pulmonary rehabilitation (see p. 86), or for assessment of their requirement for nebulized bronchodilator therapy (see p. 68) or the need for oxygen therapy (see p. 81).

Exacerbations

Exacerbations are one of the most important features of COPD. They occur in patients at all stages of their disease, but are most common in those with severe disease. Many mild exacerbations are not reported to patients' GPs,[167] but for many patients exacerbations are the only occasions when they consider themselves to have an illness and the only occasions on which they consult their GP. They manifest as worsening of existing symptoms and patients frequently believe that they have an "infection".

Exacerbations are an important determinant of adverse health status and patients can be broadly divided into those who have frequent exacerbations (three or more per year) and those who have less than three per year.[168] Most patients make a full recovery from an exacerbation within 1 week, but some patients experiencing frequent exacerbations take longer to recover and a few have not made a full recovery and their lung function

Symptoms of an exacerbation
Increased breathlessness
Increased sputum volume
Increased sputum purulence
Wheeze
Ankle swelling
Symptoms of a cold
Fever or rigors

Table 36. Symptoms of an exacerbation.

has not returned to the pre-exacerbation level by the time the next exacerbation occurs. For these patients exacerbations are an important cause of progressive deterioration.

Many exacerbations are related to infections, both viral and bacterial, but inhalation of air pollutants and changes in the weather may also be important.[169,170]

Increased breathlessness is the commonest symptom of an exacerbation. Change in sputum colour, with increased purulence, increased sputum volume and wheezing, are also common symptoms. Some patients also experience sore throats or symptoms of colds and some will develop worsening ankle swelling (Table 36).

The differential diagnosis of a worsening of symptoms includes cardiac dysfunction, pneumonia, pulmonary emboli, a pneumothorax and bronchial obstruction due to a tumour (Table 37). Without a chest radiograph it is difficult to differentiate an exacerbation of COPD from pneumonia, but in practice most of these patients will meet the criteria suggested for referral to hospital and a radiograph will be obtained.

Most patients can be managed at home but a few need hospital treatment and the BTS COPD guidelines make recommendations about factors to consider when deciding where to treat patients. Essentially, the decision involves an assessment of the severity of symptoms (particularly the degree of breathlessness, the presence of cyanosis or peripheral oedema and the level of consciousness), the presence of co-morbidities, whether or not the patient is already receiving long-term oxygen

Differential diagnosis of an exacerbation
Pulmonary embolus
Pneumothorax
Myocardial infarction
Left ventricular failure
Pneumonia
Bronchial carcinoma

Table 37. Differential diagnosis of an exacerbation.

therapy, the level of physical functioning and the patient's ability to cope at home (Table 38).

Some hospitals now operate rapid assessment units for patients referred with COPD.[171] These aim to identify those patients that can safely be managed at home with additional nursing and medical input rather than being admitted. Other hospitals operate assisted or early discharge schemes that aim to facilitate the early discharge of patients admitted with exacerbations of COPD, again by providing a package of care at home. These schemes are discussed in more detail below (p. 77).

Treatment of an exacerbation at home
The aims of treating an exacerbation are to relieve symptoms, to treat any infection that is present, to hasten recovery, and to identify patients who continue to deteriorate and who need hospital admission.

Investigations are not usually required for patients with an exacerbation of COPD managed at home. Many mild exacerbations are not reported to doctors and patients simply use more of their maintenance bronchodilators to control symptoms.[167]

Antibiotics are often prescribed to patients presenting with an exacerbation, although there is limited evidence of their efficacy.[172] The most common pathogens identified in patients at the time of exacerbations are *Haemophilus influenzae*, *Streptococcus pneumoniae* and *Moraxella catarrhalis*, but these

Factors favouring referral to hospital for management of an exacerbation
Unable to cope at home
Severe breathlessness
Poor physical function
Cyanosed
Severe peripheral oedema
Impaired consciousness
On long-term O_2 therapy (LTOT)
Rapid rate of onset

Table 38. Factors favouring referral to hospital for management of an exacerbation.

organisms can also be isolated from the sputum of patients with stable disease and their role in causing exacerbations is still unclear.[173,174] Other pathogens, such as *Chlamydia pneumoniae*, may also be important.

Few trials of antibiotic therapy have been placebo-controlled, and few have controlled for the effect of steroid administration or have studied sufficient numbers of patients. Meta-analyses have suggested a small, and probably clinically insignificant, benefit of antibiotic therapy.[175,176] On the basis of current evidence it is impossible to make firm recommendations for or against the use of antibiotics.[177] The best study supporting the use of antibiotics suggested that they were of greatest value in patients experiencing all three features of an exacerbation: increased breathlessness, increased sputum volume and increased sputum purulence;[178] they may also be appropriate if patients have at least two of these features.

Antibiotic choice will depend on local policies, but in general amoxicillin (500 mg tds), clarithromycin (500 mg bd) or trimethoprim (200 mg bd) is adequate for most patients. Patients do not usually require more than 7 days' therapy. Patients having frequent exacerbations should be given a reserve course of antibiotics to keep at home so that they may start them without delay.

Increased breathlessness can usually be managed by adding a short-acting beta agonist or anticholinergic bronchodilator, if the patient is not already receiving these, or by increasing the frequency of existing bronchodilator therapy.

Most patients can be managed using conventional inhalers, but a few benefit from nebulized therapy. Whether this is simply due to the larger doses of bronchodilator drugs that are delivered to the airways or whether it is a response to the cooling or moistening effects of the nebulizer is not clear. Deposition of drugs from a nebulizer is also less dependent on inspiratory effort. Unlike stable COPD, there is little evidence that nebulizing a combination of anticholinergic and beta agonist bronchodilators during an exacerbation improves symptoms or the rate of recovery compared with using a beta agonist alone.[179] Most patients requiring a nebulizer can be managed with 2.5 mg salbutamol given 4–6 hourly for 24–48 hours. Some will need it for longer.

Oral corticosteroids have been shown to speed recovery, shorten in-patient stays and delay the time to the next exacerbation in patients admitted to hospital with exacerbations of COPD. They appear to have a similar effects in patients managed in the community,[168,180] but are not necessary for the majority of mild exacerbations unless the increased airflow limitation fails to respond to increased bronchodilator therapy, or the patient is already on maintenance oral steroid therapy. Most patients requiring steroid therapy respond to 30 mg prednisolone daily for 7–10 days.

Patients who develop peripheral oedema at the time of an exacerbation respond to diuretic therapy, but it is important to monitor serum potassium levels, particularly if they are also receiving high dose beta agonist therapy.

Mucolytics are not usually prescribed in the UK or North America. Unlike the evidence regarding their use in stable disease, randomized controlled trials have shown that there is no benefit from adding mucolytic drugs to conventional therapy at times of exacerbations.

In addition to these specific therapies, patients should be encouraged to maintain an adequate fluid intake and to avoid sedative and hypnotic drugs.

Patients with mild exacerbations need not be reviewed unless their symptoms worsen, but those with more severe exacerbations should be reviewed within 48 hours. If they are no better, corticosteroids should be added if they were not prescribed initially and patients should be reviewed again within 48 hours, otherwise referral to hospital should be considered (see Table 39).

Management of an exacerbation in hospital

In many respects, the management of exacerbations in hospitals is similar to home management and sometimes the principal reason for admission is because the patient would be unable to manage at home. These are the patients who have been

Drug therapy for exacerbations at home

Antibiotics
Increased bronchodilators (beta-2 and anticholinergics)
Oral steroids
Diuretics

Table 39. Drug therapy for exacerbations at home.

successfully managed with hospital at home, or early or assisted discharge schemes.

History and examination When taking the history the following points should be recorded: the patient's best recent exercise tolerance; current therapy; time course and symptoms of the recent deterioration; social situation and the presence of carers at home; previous admissions; and an adequate smoking history (particularly if this is a first presentation).

Relevant signs include pyrexia, purulent sputum, wheezing, tachypnoea, use of accessory muscles, peripheral oedema, cyanosis and drowsiness.

Investigations Patients admitted to hospital should have an urgent chest radiograph (looking principally for evidence of a pneumothorax or pneumonia). Their arterial blood gas tensions should be measured and the inspired oxygen concentration recorded. They should subsequently have a full blood count and urea and electrolyte measurements, an ECG and sputum should be sent for culture if it looks purulent (Table 40).

Drug therapy Bronchodilator therapy is the mainstay of in-patient treatment. Most patients receive nebulized therapy, principally because it is more convenient to administer.[166] However, formal studies have not consistently shown an advantage for nebulized therapy compared with inhalers. Bronchodilators should be given on arrival and at frequent intervals thereafter. For moderate exacerbations either

Investigations required in patients admitted to hospital

Immediate
    Chest radiograph
    Arterial blood gases
Subsequently
    Full blood count
    Urea and electrolytes
    ECG
    Sputum for culture if it looks purulent

Table 40. Investigations required in patients admitted to hospital.

salbutamol (2.5 mg) or ipratropium (500 µg) may be used. There is again no evidence that combining beta agonists with anticholinergics is any more effective than either drug alone, but in practice combination therapy is often used, particularly for patients with severe exacerbations.

Many patients are hypoxaemic when admitted and controlled oxygen therapy should be used to achieve a PaO_2 of at least 6.6 kPa without a significant rise in the $PaCO_2$ or the development of significant acidaemia (pH <7.26). Until the arterial blood gas tensions are known, patients should receive 24% or 28% oxygen via a Venturi mask. Once the blood gas tensions are known, oxygen therapy should be adjusted accordingly. It is not uncommon to find significant hypercapnia in patients brought in by ambulance as a result of high concentration oxygen therapy during transfer, and stabilization with an appropriate FiO_2 often allows the patient to correct this themselves. If the patient is hypercapnic or acidotic the blood gas measurement must be repeated within 1 hour to determine whether the values are stable, improving or deteriorating. If the patient is not hypercapnic the adequacy of oxygenation can be assessed with pulse oximetry.

If patients develop respiratory failure ventilatory support should be considered. It is now recognized that this is best administered non-invasively (see p. 78), but where such services are not available patients may require intubation. The outcome of patients requiring intermittent positive pressure ventilation (IPPV) is better than generally thought, particularly by anaesthetists, and misconceptions about the difficulty of weaning patients or about long-term survival should not be allowed to affect the decision about intubation. When considering assisted ventilation the patient's previous exercise tolerance and quality of life, and the presence of co-morbidities, must be considered.

Antibiotic use in exacerbations of COPD is controversial, but some studies have shown benefits. The BTS COPD guidelines recommend that antibiotics should be given if two of the following three features are present: increased breathlessness, increased sputum volume or increased sputum purulence.[2]

Placebo-controlled trials have shown that systemic steroid therapy leads to more rapid improvement in FEV_1, shorter hospital stays, and delays relapse in both in-patients and out-patients with exacerbations of COPD.[180–182] Two weeks' treatment is as effective as 8 and oral therapy is as effective as intravenous. Whether these data are relevant to patients with milder exacerbations treated at home is not known.

Steroids should be discontinued after the acute episode unless the patient has shown a clear response that has not reached a plateau. In this case steroid therapy should be continued until maximum improvement has been achieved, when oral steroids should be withdrawn if possible.

Patients should be given diuretics if the venous pressure is elevated or if there is peripheral or pulmonary oedema.

Post-mortem studies have shown that pulmonary emboli are common in patients with COPD and, unless there are contraindications, immobile patients should receive appropriate prophylaxis (see Table 41 for a summary).

Home care In response to the growing pressures on hospital beds in the UK, and in recognition of the facts that patients are at risk of developing complications in hospital, and that some admissions occur simply because the patient lacks adequate support at home, home care and assisted discharge schemes have been developed.[171,183–185] These either take the form of a full assessment of the patient at the hospital by a multidisciplinary

Drug management of exacerbations

Bronchodilators
Controlled oxygen therapy
Oral steroids
Antibiotics
Diuretics
Thromboembolus prophylaxis

Table 41. Drug management of exacerbations.

team, and discharge to the community, with appropriate support or identification of patients who have been admitted to hospital at an early stage of their admission and who could be discharged before they have fully recovered with increased support. In both cases the increased support takes the form of additional equipment (e.g. a nebulizer and compressor or an oxygen concentrator), nursing supervision from visiting respiratory nurse specialists and increased social service input. Patients remain under the care of the hospital consultant, but GPs are made aware of the fact that they are receiving home care.

Assisted discharge schemes do reduce the number of days spent in hospital, but the duration of support they receive may be longer than if they had remained in hospital and some will require re-admission. Health status is better in patients treated at home,[186] but the schemes are expensive.[187] Most reports on the implementation of such schemes have come from urban areas, and they may be more difficult and more expensive to operate in dispersed rural populations.

Non-invasive ventilation In the absence of other organ system failure, and provided that the patient does not have large volumes of secretions and is able to cooperate, non-invasive ventilation (NIV) is now considered the treatment of choice for patients with hypercapnic respiratory failure (Figure 29).[188] This is usually delivered via a mask that covers the nose, but occasionally a full face mask covering the nose and the mouth is required. Patients treated with NIV are less likely to need intubation, and mortality rates are reduced.[189]

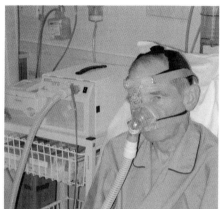

Figure 29. A patient using non-invasive ventilation during an exacerbation of COPD.

Contraindications to NIV
Coma or confusion
Inability to protect the airway
Severe acidosis at presentation
Copious respiratory secretions
Significant comorbidity
Vomiting
Obstructed bowel
Haemodynamic instability
Radiological evidence of consolidation
Orofacial abnormalities which interfere with the mask/face interface

Table 42. contraindications to NIV.

NIV may be used as: a holding measure, to assist ventilation in patients at an earlier stage than that at which intubation would be considered; as a trial, with a view to intubation if it fails; or as the ceiling of treatment in patients who are not candidates for intubation. NIV may be performed in an ITU or on a general ward.[190] The outcome of patients who remain acidotic (pH <7.30) after initial treatment is less good and these patients are best managed in a high dependency setting by experienced clinicians. The absolute or relative contraindications to the use of NIV are shown in Table 42.

Doxapram may help to get a patient through an episode of acute respiratory failure due to a reversible cause if NIV is not available.[191]

Palliative care

Once it is clear that a patient is in the terminal stages of their disease, adequate symptom palliation is essential. Non-pharmacological approaches, including counselling, breathing retraining, relaxation and teaching of coping strategies, can help.[192]

Anxiety can be controlled using buspirone, which does not suppress respiration,[193] or benzodiazepines. If rapid control is required, lorazepam (0.5–2 mg sublingually) is effective. Diazepam (5–10 mg daily) is appropriate to maintain control.

Breathlessness can be controlled using opiates (e.g. 2.5 mg diamorphine every 4 hours). If patients are unable to swallow, drug treatment can be continued using a subcutaneous infusion administered using a syringe driver (Table 43).

Palliative care
Benzodiazepines to control anxiety
Opiates to control breathlessness
Consider continuous subcutaneous infusion therapy

Table 43. Palliative care.

Other Treatment Modalities

Vaccination

Although there have been no studies specifically in patients with COPD, vaccination of patients with chronic respiratory disease against influenza has been shown to reduce hospital attendance, admission rates and death rates from influenza.[194–196] Annual influenza vaccination is recommended for all patients with COPD.[197,198]

It is now also common to vaccinate patients against the pneumococcus using the polyvalent capsular polysaccharide vaccine.[199] This has been shown to reduce the incidence of invasive pneumococcal disease in patients with chronic lung disease[200] and to be cost effective.[194]

Oxygen

As the COPD progresses many patients become hypoxaemic. In some, the rate of decline in PaO_2 can be as great as 1 kPa per year. Many patients tolerate mild hypoxaemia well, but once the resting PaO_2 falls below 8 kPa patients begin to develop signs of cor pulmonale, principally peripheral oedema. Once this occurs the prognosis is poor and if untreated the 5-year survival is less than 50%.

Long-term oxygen therapy (LTOT)

Widespread use of oxygen therapy followed the publication of data showing survival benefits from oxygen therapy in patients with severe hypoxaemia (PaO_2 <8 kPa).[201,202] Benefits were seen in patients with a normal or elevated $PaCO_2$, and in patients who had, and had not, had episodes of oedema. The greatest benefits were seen in patients receiving oxygen 19 hours per day followed by those receiving 15 hours/day. Patients receiving only 12 hours/day had only marginal benefit.

As well as the effects on survival (Figure 30), LTOT leads to less polycythaemia, reduced progression of pulmonary hypertension and improvements in neuropsychological health

(Table 44), but it has only a small beneficial effect on health status. LTOT offers no survival benefit for patients with less severe hypoxia and continuing smoking may negate the benefits of LTOT.[203]

Based on these studies, current guidelines recommend that LTOT is prescribed for patients with COPD who, *when stable*, have a resting PaO_2 <7.3 kPa, or between 7.3 and 8.0 kPa, and at least one of the following: secondary polycythaemia, nocturnal hypoxia, peripheral oedema or evidence of pulmonary

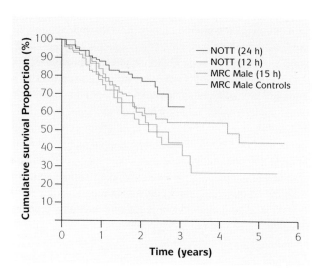

Figure 30. The effects of long-term oxygen therapy on survival in patients with COPD (based on data from Refs 201 and 202).

Benefits of LTOT
Improved long-term survival
Prevention of deterioration in pulmonary hypertension
Reduction of polycythaemia
Improved sleep quality
Increased renal blood flow
Reduction in cardiac arrhythmias

Table 44. Benefits of LTOT.

hypertension (Table 45).[2,204] To get full benefit, patients must use LTOT for at least 15 hours a day, but patients may get additional benefits from using it for longer periods. CO_2 retention may preclude oxygen therapy in some patients with COPD. Depression of the hypoxic drive to breathe leads to hypercapnia, acidosis and CO_2 narcosis. Some CO_2 retention is tolerable and, depending on the initial value, rises in the $PaCO_2$ of up to 1 kPa may be safe. No patient should receive LTOT without specialist assessment and recommendation.

Long-term oxygen is sometimes difficult for patients to accept: once started, it is likely to be lifelong. It is important to emphasize that it is not addictive and does not limit mobility around the home.

LTOT is usually provided from oxygen concentrators (Figure 31). These draw ambient oxygen into the unit and pass it through a molecular sieve that adsorbs nitrogen to leave high concentration oxygen that is delivered to the patient.

Concentrators can be prescribed by GPs in England and Wales and chest physicians in Scotland. Once a prescription has been written it usually takes 3 or 4 days for the concentrator to be installed. The prescription must specify the oxygen flow rate required, the minimum number of hours per day the patient is to use the oxygen and whether patients should be supplied

Indicators for referral for LTOT assessment
Severe COPD (FEV$_1$ <40% predicted normal)
Evidence of hypoxia
Cyanosis
Polycythaemia (raised haematocrit)
Confusion or disorientation during acute infection
Arterial oxygen saturation <92% on pulse oximeter
Documented arterial blood gas PaO_2 <7.3kPa
Evidence of right heart failure
Peripheral oedema (ankle swelling)
Raised jugular venous pressure
Weight gain due to fluid retention

Table 45. Indicators for referral for LTOT assessment.

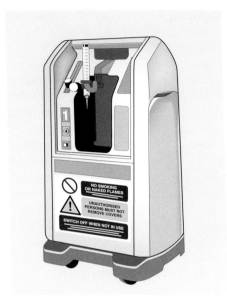

Figure 31. An oxygen concentrator.

with a fixed performance mask (i.e. one that delivers a fixed concentration of oxygen) or nasal cannulae. Nasal cannulae are the most commonly used delivery devices; they are simple to use and are generally comfortable, allowing eating and talking as normal. Humidification of low flows (1–3 l/min) of oxygen through face masks and nasal cannulae is not recommended.

Fire and explosion are real dangers and there have been many reports of patients starting fires, usually by lighting a cigarette whilst wearing nasal cannulae.[205] Patients and their families and carers must be warned not to smoke in the vicinity of the oxygen.

The benefits of supplemental oxygen for patients who are not hypoxic during the day but who have nocturnal desaturation (SaO_2 <90% for more than 30% of the night) are less clear. These patients are relatively common, but they do not appear to gain any survival advantage from nocturnal oxygen therapy and treatment does not delay the need for LTOT.[95–97]

Ambulatory oxygen therapy

Other forms of oxygen therapy are also available, but their benefits are less clear-cut. Ambulatory oxygen therapy provides portable oxygen during exercise and activities of daily living, whilst short burst (intermittent) oxygen therapy relieves breathlessness.

Ambulatory oxygen therapy can improve exercise tolerance,[206–208] quality of life and compliance with LTOT. Patients derive variable benefits and these cannot be predicted from baseline exercise capacity or lung function impairment. There are no agreed criteria for ambulatory oxygen therapy, but patients who desaturate on exercise (a fall of at least 4% below 90%), have a $\geq 10\%$ improvement in exercise capacity and are motivated to use the oxygen outside the house, may benefit from ambulatory oxygen therapy.[204]

Currently, ambulatory oxygen therapy in the UK is usually provided from small (230 l) cylinders. These have a limited capacity, providing only 2 hours at 2 l/min, and cannot be refilled in the patient's home. Oxygen-conserving devices, which restrict the flow of oxygen to the inspiratory phase of respiration, have been developed.[209] These can prolong the effective life of the cylinder, but are not prescribable in the UK.

Ambulatory oxygen can also be supplied from canisters containing liquid oxygen.[210] These can supply 4 hours of oxygen at 4 l/min. Liquid oxygen is more expensive than gaseous oxygen and is also not currently available in the UK.

Intermittent oxygen therapy

Intermittent oxygen therapy is commonly prescribed for use by patients who do not meet the criteria for LTOT. The principal indication is breathlessness, often following exertion, which is relieved by oxygen and which is associated with a fall in SaO_2. There are no guidelines about the use of such treatment and no data to support or refute its use, but many patients do appear to benefit.

Pulmonary rehabilitation

Pulmonary rehabilitation is an increasingly popular and effective option for patients with moderate to severe COPD. Rehabilitation aims to prevent deconditioning and allow the patient to cope with their disease. Most programmes are hospital based and comprise individualized exercise programmes and educational talks, but a major component is the sharing of experiences amongst participants and their spouses. Pulmonary rehabilitation can reduce symptoms, increase mobility, improve quality of life[211,212] and it may also reduce hospital re-admission rates.

Programmes are widely available in North America and Europe, but availability is still limited in the UK. The detailed content of the programmes varies considerably, but this seems to have little effect on outcomes.[212] Programmes based in secondary care are effective, but may suffer from a high dropout rate and patients may be deterred from attending by the frequent journeys to the hospital.[213] Those based in the home may be less effective because patients do not perform the prescribed exercises and miss the group therapy aspects of hospital-based programmes. There is now growing interest in running programmes in primary care.

There are no specific referral criteria, but patients must be sufficiently mobile and motivated to attend the programme (see Tables 46 and 47).[214]

Essential components of pulmonary rehabilitation program

Exercise training
Education about:
  The disease and its management
  Benefits and financial support available
  Travel
Psychological and behavioural interventions
Outcome assessment

Table 46. Essential components of pulmonary rehabilitation programmes.

Even if a formal pulmonary rehabilitation programme is not available locally, patients can help themselves by undertaking exercise at home. They should be advised to do some exercise each day and to set realistic goals (Table 48).

Nutritional support

Many patients with COPD lose weight as a consequence of decreased food intake as a result of breathlessness, altered absorption as a result of hypoxia and increased resting energy expenditure as a result of the increased work of breathing.[215] Patients who are underweight have an increased mortality and this can be reduced by appropriate nutritional support.[86]

Benefits of pulmonary rehabilitation programmes

Increased exercise capacity
Better health status
Reduced primary care consultation rates
Reduced hospital admissions

Table 47. Benefits of pulmonary rehabilitation programmes.

Advice about exercise for patients if a rehabilitation programme is not available locally

Discuss plans with your GP
Start small
Walk every day
Pace yourself
Start during the spring and summer
Exercise consistently and set realistic goals
Educate yourself
    Ask for advice
    Read leaflets from the British Lung Foundation
    Write down questions for you GP or practice nurse
Keep exercising during winter
Keep going even during bad times
Consider joining Breathe Easy

Table 48. Advice about exercise for patients if a rehabilitation programme is not available locally.

Surgery

Lung volume reduction surgery

Over the last 50 years, many surgical interventions to improve breathlessness in patients with COPD have been tried. In general, these have been ineffective and have carried high mortality.[216] Recently, surgery to remove functionless areas of lung in patients with COPD has been shown to have benefits. This is known as lung volume reduction surgery (LVRS) and works by improving the mechanics of breathing by reducing thoracic volumes. It was initially used as a palliative procedure in patients awaiting lung transplantation, but thousands of patients have now been operated upon and striking improvements have been seen.

Lung volume reduction surgery produces clinically and statistically significant improvements in FEV_1, shuttle walking distance and quality of life,[217] but does not appear to affect mortality.

Most, but not all, patients benefit from surgery and patient selection is crucial. The indications for LVRS are severe physiological impairment (FEV_1 <35%), marked hyper-inflation and severe disability despite maximal medical therapy. Patients who have heterogeneous disease on CT are more suitable for LVRS (Table 49). Hypercapnia ($PaCO_2$ >55 mmHg) or a diffusing capacity less than 20% predicted are contraindications.[218]

Lung transplantation

Single or bilateral lung transplantation presents another option for the surgical treatment of severe emphysema. In general, transplantation is only indicated if the patient's condition has deteriorated to the point that they are severely limited and their estimated life expectancy is short.

Older patients have a significantly higher operative mortality and a worse long-term survival than younger patients,[219] and most units will not transplant patients aged over 65.

Indications for lung volume reduction surgery
Severe airflow limitation (FEV$_1$ <35%)
Hyperinflation
Severe disability
Heterogenous disease on CT

Table 49. Indications for lung volume reduction surgery.

Indications for single lung transplantation
Severe airflow limitation (FEV$_1$ <25%)
Respiratory failure (PaCO$_2$ >7.3 kPa)
Severe disability
Progressive deterioration
Pulmonary hypertension

Table 50. Indications for single lung transplantation.

Indications for transplantation are shown in Table 50. Symptomatic osteoporosis is a relative contraindication and patients with a high or low body mass index require either nutritional support or weight loss prior to transplantation. Use of low dose (<20 mg/day prednisolone) is not now considered a contraindication to transplantation.[220]

Postoperatively, there are improvements in lung function, PaO$_2$, walking distance and health status, but overall transplants do not appear to improve long-term survival. The current 5-year survival figures are around 50%.[221–223]

Psychological aspects

Many patients with COPD are depressed, often as a result of the isolation and physical limitations that their disease brings. Antidepressant drugs are frequently beneficial, but psychological assessment and therapy can also be of considerable value.

COPD and Travel

Many patients with COPD continue to want to travel. Travel within the UK is usually not a problem and oxygen concentrators can be transported in cars. Flying may present more difficulties.

Air travel

Aircraft cabins are not usually pressurized to sea level and patients with compensated COPD at sea level may experience significant hypoxaemia when flying. Patients may become breathless, wheezy or develop chest pain, and on long flights right heart failure may develop. Patients should carry their inhalers in their hand luggage. Portable nebulizers may be used in aircraft cabins, but this is at the discretion of the cabin crew.

The best predictor of the need for in-flight oxygen is the PaO_2 on the ground. Criteria for assessing the need for in-flight oxygen are shown in Table 51.

Patients on LTOT need in-flight oxygen and need to make their own provision for oxygen during waiting periods at airports. Procedures for requesting in-flight oxygen and costs differ between airlines, but most require medical authorization and at least 48 hours notice prior to departure.[224] Patients should check with the airline at the time of booking.

Assessing need for in flight oxygen	
SaO_2 >95%	Oxygen not required in flight
SaO_2 92–95%	
No additional risk factor	Oxygen not required in flight
Hypercapnia, ventilatory support, recent exacerbation, cardiac disease, cerebrovascular disease	Need a formal assessment of need for in flight oxygen
SaO_2 <92%	Need in flight oxygen

Table 51. Assessing need for in-flight oxygen.

Future Developments

The next few years are likely to see significant advances in the management of COPD. Earlier diagnosis of patients with milder disease combined with effective smoking cessation services may prevent the development of moderate and severe disease in many patients. More structured management in primary care, with regular review, and the wider availability of pulmonary rehabilitation will improve the care of patients with moderate and severe disease, and the development of new therapies offers hope for all patients. Most of the drugs currently used to treat COPD were originally developed for use in asthma. Increased interest in COPD over the last decade has led to the development of molecules specifically to treat this disease. A new bronchodilator is likely to be the first of these to make a significant impact, but over time, new anti-inflammatory therapies should also become available.

Tiotropium has already been discussed. It is a new M_1 and M_3 (see p. 63) selective long-acting anticholinergic bronchodilator[130] that has been shown to cause bronchodilatation, reduce breathlessness, improve health status and reduce exacerbation rates. It offers significant promise for patients with COPD.

Drugs which inhibit phosphodiesterase type 4 (PDE4; see p. 27) can cause bronchodilation and inhibit neutrophilic inflammation. A number of molecules are in the late stages of clinical development. They reduce breathlessness, improve health status and may also reduce exacerbations, but their use may be limited by the fact that a significant proportion of patients develop transient gastrointestinal side-effects.[225]

A number of anti-inflammatory drugs and specific mediator antagonists are in development,[226] and if they prove effective they may both improve symptoms and prevent or slow disease progression.

Drugs that reduce mucus secretion or improve mucociliary clearance are also in development. Some block the inflammatory signals that lead to increased mucus secretion whilst others inhibit mucin secretion. Intriguingly, macrolide antibiotics have been shown to act in this way,[227] and this may partially explain their actions in treating exacerbations.

Frequently Asked Questions

What is COPD?

COPD stands for **C**hronic **O**bstructive **P**ulmonary **D**isease, which is now the internationally accepted term for a lung condition that causes narrowing of the airways and damage to the lung tissue leading to coughing and breathlessness.

What are the differences between COPD and emphysema or chronic bronchitis?

COPD is a term for a condition that includes different patterns of symptoms and varying amounts of damage and inflammation in the lung. Both emphysema, which is damage to the alveoli (or air sacks) in the lung where gas exchange occurs, and chronic bronchitis, which is inflammation in the large airways leading to coughing and sputum production, are part of the range of changes seen in COPD.

What is the difference between COPD and asthma?

Both COPD and asthma are conditions associated with narrowing of the airways and airflow limitation. In asthma, the narrowing varies significantly from day to day and within a day, whereas in COPD the narrowing is relatively fixed and does not vary to any significant extent. Studies have shown that the pattern of inflammation seen in the lungs involves different cell types in asthma and COPD.

How common is COPD?

It is difficult to know how common COPD really is, as many patients with mild disease do not consult their doctor. The best estimates are that it affects at least one in ten adults aged over 40.

What causes COPD?

The most important cause of COPD in western countries is smoking. Some cases occur as a result of breathing in certain dusts at work, and a few are due to an inherited increased susceptibility to the effects of inhaled noxious dusts and chemicals.

Do all smokers develop COPD?

No. Between one in five and one in three will develop symptoms of COPD. More show evidence of asymptomatic narrowing of the airways if tested. What determines whether people are affected or not is still not understood. The number of cigarettes smoked is important and people who start smoking early seem more likely to develop COPD. This is particularly true for women. Genetic factors also seem important.

Are all forms of smoking equally bad?

COPD can be caused by smoking manufactured and self-rolled cigarettes, cigars and pipe tobacco, but there is some evidence that cigars and pipe tobacco are slightly less likely to cause COPD.

Will I get better?

Unfortunately, the damage caused to the lungs in COPD does not go away. Stopping smoking prevents the accelerated decline in lung function seen in smokers, but so far no treatment has been shown to affect the progression of the disease.

Can anything be done to prevent COPD?

COPD is very uncommon in non-smokers and in people who are not exposed to passive cigarette smoke. Avoiding smoking and wearing adequate respiratory protection (i.e. masks) if working in dusty occupations are the best ways of preventing COPD.

What are the symptoms of COPD?

The commonest symptoms are breathlessness on exertion (e.g. climbing hills or stairs), a cough (which may be productive of white or green sputum) and exacerbations (which may appear to be chest infections or episodes of bronchitis and which often occur in the winter). Other symptoms are wheezing, chest pain, ankle swelling, weight loss and feeling depressed.

What is an exacerbation?

Exacerbations are periods when existing symptoms of COPD worsen, medications appear to be less effective or new symptoms develop. Many patients feel that they have a chest infection and indeed some exacerbations are caused by infection, particularly viral infections, but others may be triggered by dusts that are inhaled or changes in the weather.

How is COPD diagnosed?

COPD is often diagnosed solely on the basis of a patient's symptoms and the fact that they have smoked. To make an accurate diagnosis of COPD it is necessary to show that there is narrowing of the airways and that the narrowing does not change much either from day to day or in response to treatment. This is best done by performing a breathing test called spirometry before and after a trial of treatment.

What is spirometry?

Spirometry is a way of measuring the amount of air exhaled from the lungs. It is usual to measure the total amount of air exhaled after taking in as deep a breath as possible (this is known as the vital capacity or VC). The exhalation is usually done using maximum effort, in which case the amount of air exhaled is known as the forced vital capacity (FVC), but it can also be done gently, in which case the amount exhaled is known as the slow vital capacity (slow VC). Spirometry also measures the amount of air exhaled in the first second (this is known as the forced expiratory volume in 1 second or FEV_1). If there is narrowing of the airways, less air is exhaled in the first second and so the FEV_1, and the FEV_1 as a proportion of the FVC, are reduced.

How is COPD treated?

The treatment for COPD depends on what symptoms are present and how extensive the damage to the lungs is. Many patients only need treatment at the time of an exacerbation and this is often simply a course of antibiotics. Patients with regular symptoms usually need to inhale drugs that relax the muscle in the walls of the airways and reduce the narrowing that is present. Patients who have severe narrowing of the airways and who are having frequent exacerbations may also be prescribed a steroid inhaler to try to reduce the frequency of exacerbations. In more advanced cases, patients may be given extra oxygen to breathe either in short bursts to relieve symptoms or continuously for at least 16 hours per day. Some patients need courses of steroid tablets at the time of an exacerbation and a few are prescribed regular steroid tablets.

Do I have to have steroids?

Inhaled steroids have been shown to reduce the frequency of exacerbations in patients with advanced COPD. Their role in milder disease is less clear. Steroid tablets have been shown to speed the recovery of patients admitted to hospital with an exacerbation and delay the development of future exacerbations. They appear to have similar benefits when used to treat exacerbations in patients not admitted to hospital. Their benefits when used as regular, daily treatment are less clear, but some patients do seem to derive benefit and appear to deteriorate if the dose is reduced or if the tablets are stopped.

Can I keep doing the things I have been doing?

COPD causes breathlessness on exertion and as the disease progresses it gets harder for patients to do the things they have been used to doing at the same speed. They may still be able to do some things but at a slower pace, but they may find that their breathlessness eventually prevents them from doing some things that they have been used to doing. However, it is important to try to keep physically active, as this seems to reduce the impact of the lung damage and enables patients to keep doing more for longer.

Should I be on a special diet?

There is no evidence that specific diets are beneficial for patients with COPD, but it is important that patients are not overweight, as this may worsen their breathlessness on exertion. Some patients with advanced disease lose weight as part of the illness and this may lead to weakness of the chest muscles.

These patients need to maintain an adequate calorie intake. Patients who produce significant amounts of sputum observe that the amount of sputum is reduced and it is easier to cough it up if they reduce the amount of dairy produce in their diet. The reason for this is not known.

Can I still go on holiday?

Many patients with COPD continue to travel. Some patients may need to arrange for oxygen to be available on aircraft and may need wheelchair assistance at airports or train stations. Patients should always ensure that they take adequate supplies of all their medications with them and that they have appropriate insurance.

Do I need a nebulizer?

Nebulizers are simply devices that deliver high doses of drugs to the lung in a mist form. They are operated by air from a compressor. Most patients can be treated using inhalers, but a few benefit from the higher doses of drugs and some may also benefit from the cooling effect of the particles and the fact that less effort is needed to inhale the drugs than if inhalers are used.

Do I need oxygen?

As COPD progresses, the level of oxygen in the blood falls. In some patients this fall puts a strain on the heart and unless treated with oxygen their condition rapidly worsens. These patients need to breathe oxygen for at least 16 hours each day. In patients with less severe disease, oxygen levels sometimes fall during exertion and some of these patients are able to do more if they breathe oxygen during exertion. All patients being considered for oxygen therapy need careful assessment, as oxygen can be harmful to some patients.

Should I have a flu vaccination?

It is a good idea for all patients with COPD to have an annual influenza vaccination unless they have previous allergic reactions to the vaccine.

Should I try to exercise?

Regular exercise within the limitations imposed by breathlessness maintains fitness and reduces disability. Even patients who have not been used to taking any exercise can benefit from graded exercises, particularly when part of a pulmonary rehabilitation programme.

Will my children develop COPD?

Almost all cases of COPD are due to smoking, but there do appear to be inherited factors which affect whether or not smokers develop COPD. If the children of a patient with COPD do not smoke they are very unlikely to develop COPD themselves.

What is α-1 antitrypsin deficiency?

α-1 Antitrypsin (AT) deficiency is an inherited condition which results in low levels of a protein known as α-1 antitrypsin. This forms part of the lung's defences against damage and patients who are deficient in α-1 antitrypsin are more likely to develop emphysema if they smoke.

Will I need to go to hospital?

Many patients with COPD are treated in the community, but some will be referred to hospital. There are a number of reasons why referrals are made and these include: the need for a specialist opinion; to have their need for oxygen or nebulized therapy assessed; or for treatment of exacerbations.

References

1. Lopez AD, Murray CC. The global burden of disease, 1990–2020. *Nat Med* 1998; **4**(11): 1241–1243.

2. COPD Guidelines Group of the Standards of Care Committee of the BTS. BTS guidelines for the management of chronic obstructive pulmonary disease. *Thorax* 1997; **52**(Suppl 5): S1–S28.

3. Samet JM. Definitions and methedology in COPD research. In: Hensley MJ, Saunders NA, editors. *Clinical Epidemiology of Chronic Obstructive Pulmonary Disease*. New York: Marcel Dekker, 1989; pp. 1–22.

4. Miller MR. Chronic obstructive pulmonary disease and '150 years of blowing'. *Hosp Med* 1998; **59**(9): 719–722.

5. CIBA Foundation Guest Symposium. Terminology, definitions and classification of chronic obstructive pulmonary emphysema and related conditions. *Thorax* 1959; **14**: 286–299.

6. Anthonisen NR, Wright EC, IPPB Trial Group. Bronchodilator response in chronic obstructive pulmonary disease. *Am Rev Respir Disease* 1986; **133**: 814–819.

7. American Thoracic Society. Standards for the diagnosis and care of patients with chronic obstructive pulmonary disease. *Am J Respir Crit Care Med* 1995; **152**(5, Pt 2): S77–S121.

8. Siafakas NM, Vermeire P, Pride NB, Paoletti P, Gibson J, Howard P *et al*. Optimal assessment and management of chronic obstructive pulmonary disease (COPD). The European Respiratory Society Task Force. *Eur Respir J* 1995; **8**(8): 1398–1420.

9. Pauwels RA, Buist AS, Calverley PM, Jenkins CR, Hurd SS. Global strategy for the diagnosis, management, and prevention of chronic obstructive pulmonary disease. NHLBI/WHO Global Initiative for Chronic Obstructive Lung Disease (GOLD) Workshop summary. *Am J Respir Crit Care Med* 2001; **163**(5): 1256–1276.

10. Eber E, Zach MS. Long term sequelae of bronchopulmonary dysplasia (chronic lung disease of infancy). *Thorax* 2001; **56**(4): 317–323.

11. Doll R, Peto R, Wheatley K, Gray R, Sutherland I. Mortality in relation to smoking: 40 years' observations on male British doctors. *Br Med J* 1994; **309**(6959): 901–911.

12. Fletcher C, Peto R, Tinker C, Speizer F. *The Natural History of Chronic Bronchitis and Emphysema. An 8 Year Study of Working Men*. Oxford: Oxford University Press, 1976.

13. Fletcher C, Peto R. The natural history of chronic airflow obstruction. *Br Med J* 1977; **1**(6077): 1645–1648.

14. Burrows B, Knudson RJ, Cline MG, Lebowitz MD. Quantitative relationships between cigarette smoking and ventilatory function. *Am Rev Respir Dis* 1977; **115**(2): 195–205.

15. Beck GJ, Doyle CA, Schachter EN. Smoking and lung function. *Am Rev Respir Dis* 1981; **123**(2): 149–155.

16. Givelber RJ, Couropmitree NN, Gottlieb DJ, Evans JC, Levy D, Myers RH *et al*. Segregation analysis of pulmonary function among families in the Framingham Study. *Am J Respir Crit Care Med* 1998; **157**(5, Pt 1): 1445–1451.

17. Redline S, Tishler PV, Lewitter FI, Tager IB, Munoz A, Speizer FE. Assessment of genetic and nongenetic influences on pulmonary function. A twin study. *Am Rev Respir Dis* 1987; **135**(1): 217–222.

18. Silverman EK. Genetics of chronic obstructive pulmonary disease. *Novartis Found Symp* 2001; **234**: 45–58; discussion 58–64.

19. Sandford AJ, Pare PD. Genetic risk factors for chronic obstructive pulmonary disease. *Clin Chest Med* 2000; **21**(4): 633–643.

20. Sluiter HJ, Koeter GH, de Monchy JG, Postma DS, de Vries K, Orie NG. The Dutch hypothesis (chronic non-specific lung disease) revisited. *Eur Respir J* 1991; **4**(4): 479–489.

21. Peto R, Speizer FE, Cochrane AL, Moore F, Fletcher CM, Tinker CM *et al*. The relevance in adults of air-flow obstruction, but not of mucus hypersecretion, to mortality from chronic lung disease. Results from 20 years of prospective observation. *Am Rev Respir Dis* 1983; **128**(3): 491–500.

22. Clement J, Van de Woestijne KP. Rapidly decreasing forced expiratory volume in one second or vital capacity and development of chronic airflow obstruction. *Am Rev Respir Dis* 1982; **125**(5): 553–558.

23. Kanner RE, Renzetti AD, Jr, Klauber MR, Smith CB, Golden CA. Variables associated with changes in spirometry in patients with obstructive lung diseases. *Am J Med* 1979; **67**(1): 44–50.

24. Lange P, Nyboe J, Appleyard M, Jensen G, Schnohr P. Relation of ventilatory impairment and of chronic mucus hypersecretion to mortality from obstructive lung disease and from all causes. *Thorax* 1990; **45**(8): 579–585.

25. Kanner RE, Anthonisen NR, Connett JE. Lower respiratory illnesses promote FEV(1) decline in current smokers but not ex-smokers with mild chronic obstructive pulmonary disease. Results from the lung health study. *Am J Respir Crit Care Med* 2001; **164**(3): 358–364.

26. Vestbo J, Prescott E, Lange P. Association of chronic mucus hypersecretion with FEV1 decline and chronic obstructive pulmonary disease morbidity. Copenhagen City Heart Study Group. *Am J Respir Crit Care Med* 1996; **153**(5): 1530–1535.

27. Seemungal TA, Donaldson GC, Bhowmik A, Jeffries DJ, Wedzicha JA. Time course and recovery of exacerbations in patients with chronic obstructive pulmonary disease. *Am J Respir Crit Care Med* 2000; **161**(5): 1608–1613.

28. Tashkin DP, Altose MD, Connett JE, Kanner RE, Lee WW, Wise RA. Methacholine reactivity predicts changes in lung function over time in smokers with early chronic obstructive pulmonary disease. The Lung Health Study Research Group. *Am J Respir Crit Care Med* 1996; **153**(6, Pt 1): 1802–1811.

29. Chen JC, Mannino DM. Worldwide epidemiology of chronic obstructive pulmonary disease. *Curr Opin Pulm Med* 1999; **5**(2): 93–99.

30. Coggon D, Newman Taylor A. Coal mining and chronic obstructive pulmonary disease: a review of the evidence. *Thorax* 1998; **53**(5): 398–407.

31. Pride NB, Connellan SJ. Chronic bronchitis in non-smokers. Introductory review. *Eur J Respir Dis Suppl* 1982; **118**: 9–14.

32. Hendrick DJ. Occupational and chronic obstructive pulmonary disease (COPD). *Thorax* 1996; **51**(9): 947–955.

33. Barker DJ, Godfrey KM, Fall C, Osmond C, Winter PD, Shaheen SO. Relation of birth weight and childhood respiratory infection to adult lung function and death from chronic obstructive airways disease. *Br Med J* 1991; **303**(6804): 671–675.

34. Shaheen S, Barker DJ. Early lung growth and chronic airflow obstruction. *Thorax* 1994; **49**(6): 533–536.

35. Shahar E, Folsom AR, Melnick SL, Tockman MS, Comstock GW, Gennaro V *et al*. Dietary $n-3$ polyunsaturated fatty acids and smoking-related chronic obstructive pulmonary disease. Atherosclerosis Risk in Communities Study Investigators. *New Engl J Med* 1994; **331**(4): 228–233.

36. Britton JR, Pavord ID, Richards KA, Knox AJ, Wisniewski AF, Lewis SA *et al*. Dietary antioxidant vitamin intake and lung function in the general population. *Am J Respir Crit Care Med* 1995; **151**(5): 1383–1387.

37. Carrell RW, Jeppsson JO, Laurell CB, Brennan SO, Owen MC, Vaughan L *et al*. Structure and variation of human alpha 1-antitrypsin. *Nature* 1982; **298**(5872): 329–334.

38. Laurell CB, Eriksson S. The electrophoretic alpha-1 globulin pattern of serum in alpha-1-antitrypsin deficiency. *Scand J Clin Lab Invest* 1963; **15**: 133–140.

39. Eriksson S. A 30-year perspective on alpha 1-antitrypsin deficiency. *Chest* 1996; **110**(6, Suppl): 237S–242S.

40. Lieberman J, Gaidulis L, Garoutte B, Mittman C. Identification and characteristics of the common Alpha 1-antitrypsin phenotypes. *Chest* 1972; **62**(5): 557–564.

41. Tobin MJ, Cook PJ, Hutchison DC. Alpha 1 antitrypsin deficiency: the clinical and physiological features of pulmonary emphysema in subjects homozygous for Pi type Z. A survey by the British Thoracic Association. *Br J Dis Chest* 1983; **77**(1): 14–27.

42. Turino GM, Barker AF, Brantly ML, Cohen AB, Connelly RP, Crystal RG *et al*. Clinical features of individuals with PI*SZ phenotype of alpha 1-antitrypsin deficiency. Alpha 1-Antitrypsin Deficiency Registry Study Group. *Am J Respir Crit Care Med* 1996; **154**(6, Pt 1): 1718–1725.

43. Cox DW, Levison H. Emphysema of early onset associated with a complete deficiency of alpha-1-antitrypsin (null homozygotes). *Am Rev Respir Dis* 1988; **137**(2): 371–375.

44. Seersholm N, Kok-Jensen A, Dirksen A. Survival of patients with severe alpha 1-antitrypsin deficiency with special reference to non-index cases. *Thorax* 1994; **49**(7): 695–698.

45. Hutchison DC. Alpha 1-antitrypsin deficiency in Europe: geographical distribution of Pi types S and Z. *Respir Med* 1998; **92**(3): 367–377.

46. Hutchison DC. Alpha 1-Proteinase inhibitor deficiency. In: Brewis RAL, Corrin B, Geddes DM, Gibson GJ, editors. *Respiratory Medicine*. London: W. B. Saunders, 1995; pp. 1034–1041.

47. Office for National Statistics. *Mortality Statistics: Cause, 1999*. DH2 (No. 26). London: HMSO, 2000.

48. Anderson RH, Esmail A, Hollowell J *et al*. *Epidemiologically Based Needs Assessment: Lower Respiratory Disease*. London: HMSO, 1994.

49. Office of Population Census and Surveys. *Morbidity Statistics from General Practice. Fourth National Study 1991–1992*. London: HMSO, 1995.

50. Cox BD. Blood pressure and respiratory function. In: *The Health and Lifestyle Survey*. Preliminary report of a nationwide survey of the physical and mental health, attitudes and lifestyle of a random sample of 9,003 British adults. London: Health Promotion Research Trust, 1987; pp. 17–33.

51. Seamark DA, Williams S, Timon S, Ward A, Ward D, Seamark C *et al*. Home or surgery based screening for chronic obstructive pulmonary disease (COPD)? *Prim Care Respir J* 2001; **10**(2): 30–33.

52. Higgins MW, Thom T. Incidence, prevalence and mortality: intra- and intercountry differences. In: Hensley M, Saunders NA, editors. *Clinical Epidemiology of Chronic Obstructive Pulmonary Disease*. New York: Marcel Dekker, 1989; pp. 23–42.

53. Bang KM. Prevalence of chronic obstructive pulmonary disease in blacks. *J Natl Med Assoc* 1993; **85**(1): 51–55.

54. Mannino DM, Brown C, Giovino GA. Obstructive lung disease deaths in the United States from 1979 through 1993. An analysis using multiple-cause mortality data. *Am J Respir Crit Care Med* 1997; **156**(3, Pt 1): 814–818.

55. Office for National Statistics. *Health Statistics Quarterly*, No. 8, Winter 2000. London: HMSO, 2000.

56. Saetta M, Turato G, Maestrelli P, Mapp CE, Fabbri LM. Cellular and structural bases of chronic obstructive pulmonary disease. *Am J Respir Crit Care Med* 2001; **163**(6): 1304–1309.

57. Magee F, Wright JL, Wiggs BR, Pare PD, Hogg JC. Pulmonary vascular structure and function in chronic obstructive pulmonary disease. *Thorax* 1988; **43**(3): 183–189.

58. Agusti AG. Systemic effects of chronic obstructive pulmonary disease. *Novartis Found Symp* 2001; **234**: 242–249; discussion 250–254.

59. Turato G, Di Stefano A, Maestrelli P, Mapp CE, Ruggieri MP, Roggeri A *et al*. Effect of smoking cessation on airway inflammation in chronic bronchitis. *Am J Respir Crit Care Med* 1995; **152**(4, Pt 1): 1262–1267.

60. Rutgers SR, Postma DS, ten Hacken NH, Kauffman HF, van Der Mark TW, Koeter GH *et al*. Ongoing airway inflammation in patients with COPD who do not currently smoke. *Thorax* 2000; **55**(1): 12–18.

61. Hogg JC, Macklem PT, Thurlbeck WM. Site and nature of airway obstruction in chronic obstructive lung disease. *New Engl J Med* 1968; **278**(25): 1355–1360.

62. Saetta M, Ghezzo H, Kim WD, King M, Angus GE, Wang NS *et al*. Loss of alveolar attachments in smokers. A morphometric correlate of lung function impairment. *Am Rev Respir Dis* 1985; **132**(4): 894–900.

63. Shapiro SD. Evolving concepts in the pathogenesis of chronic obstructive pulmonary disease. *Clin Chest Med* 2000; **21**(4): 621–632.

64. Niewoehner DE, Kleinerman J, Rice DB. Pathologic changes in the peripheral airways of young cigarette smokers. *New Engl J Med* 1974; **291**(15): 755–758.

65. Saetta M, Baraldo S, Corbino L, Turato G, Braccioni F, Rea F *et al*. CD8+ve cells in the lungs of smokers with chronic obstructive pulmonary disease. *Am J Respir Crit Care Med* 1999; **160**(2): 711–717.

66. O'Shaughnessy TC, Ansari TW, Barnes NC, Jeffery PK. Inflammation in bronchial biopsies of subjects with chronic bronchitis: inverse relationship of CD8+ T lymphocytes with FEV1. *Am J Respir Crit Care Med* 1997; **155**(3): 852–857.

67. MacNee W, Wiggs B, Belzberg AS, Hogg JC. The effect of cigarette smoking on neutrophil kinetics in human lungs. *New Engl J Med* 1989; **321**(14): 924–928.

68. Jeffery PK. Structural and inflammatory changes in COPD: a comparison with asthma. *Thorax* 1998; **53**(2): 129–136.

69. Saetta M, Di Stefano A, Maestrelli P, Turato G, Ruggieri MP, Roggeri A *et al*. Airway eosinophilia in chronic bronchitis during exacerbations. *Am J Respir Crit Care Med* 1994; **150**(6, Pt 1): 1646–1652.

70. Shapiro SD. The macrophage in chronic obstructive pulmonary disease. *Am J Respir Crit Care Med* 1999; **160**(5, Pt 2): S29–S32.

71. Williams TJ, Jose PJ. Neutrophils in chronic obstructive pulmonary disease. *Novartis Found Symp* 2001; **234**: 136–141; discussion 141–148.

72. Hubbard RC, Fells G, Gadek J, Pacholok S, Humes J, Crystal RG. Neutrophil accumulation in the lung in alpha 1-antitrypsin deficiency. Spontaneous release of leukotriene B4 by alveolar macrophages. *J Clin Invest* 1991; **88**(3): 891–897.

73. Stockley RA. Neutrophils and protease/antiprotease imbalance. *Am J Respir Crit Care Med* 1999; **160**(5, Pt 2): S49–S52.

74. Torphy TJ. Phosphodiesterase isozymes: molecular targets for novel antiasthma agents. *Am J Respir Crit Care Med* 1998; **157**(2): 351–370.

75. Barnes PJ. Mechanisms in COPD: differences from asthma. *Chest* 2000; **117**(2, Suppl): 10S–4S.

76. Gibson GJ. Pulmonary hyperinflation: a clinical overview. *Eur Respir J* 1996; **9**(12): 2640–2649.

77. Begin P, Grassino A. Inspiratory muscle dysfunction and chronic hypercapnia in chronic obstructive pulmonary disease. *Am Rev Respir Dis* 1991; **143**(5, Pt 1): 905–912.

78. MacNee W. Pathophysiology of cor pulmonale in chronic obstructive pulmonary disease. Part One. *Am J Respir Crit Care Med* 1994; **150**(3): 833–852.

79. Harris P, Heath D. The pulmonary vasculature in emphysema. In: Harris P, Heath D, editors. *The Human Pulmonary Circulation*. Edinburgh: Churchill Livingstone, 1986; pp. 507–521.

80. Bignon J, Khoury F, Even P, Andre J, Brouet G. Morphometric study in chronic obstructive bronchopulmonary disease. Pathologic, clinical, and physiologic correlations. *Am Rev Respir Dis* 1969; **99**(5): 669–695.

81. Calverley P. Ventilatory control and dyspnea. In: Calverley P, Pride N, editors. *Chronic Obstructive Pulmonary Disease*. London: Chapman & Hall, 1995; pp. 205–242.

82. Sassoon CS, Hassell KT, Mahutte CK. Hyperoxic-induced hypercapnia in stable chronic obstructive pulmonary disease. *Am Rev Respir Dis* 1987; **135**(4): 907–911.

83. Aubier M, Murciano D, Milic-Emili J, Touaty E, Daghfous J, Pariente R *et al*. Effects of the administration of O_2 on ventilation and blood gases in patients with chronic obstructive pulmonary disease during acute respiratory failure. *Am Rev Respir Dis* 1980; **122**(5): 747–754.

84. Crossley DJ, McGuire GP, Barrow PM, Houston PL. Influence of inspired oxygen concentration on deadspace, respiratory drive, and $PaCO_2$ in intubated patients with chronic obstructive pulmonary disease. *Crit Care Med* 1997; **25**(9): 1522–1526.

85. Nunn JF, Milledge JS, Chen D, Dore C. Respiratory criteria of fitness for surgery and anaesthesia. *Anaesthesia* 1988; **43**(7): 543–551.

86. Schols AM, Slangen J, Volovics L, Wouters EF. Weight loss is a reversible factor in the prognosis of chronic obstructive pulmonary disease. *Am J Respir Crit Care Med* 1998; **157**(6, Pt 1): 1791–1797.

87. Zielinski J, Bednarek M. Early detection of COPD in a high-risk population using spirometric screening. *Chest* 2001; **119**(3): 731–736.

88. Warner KE. Cost effectiveness of smoking-cessation therapies. Interpretation of the evidence – and implications for coverage. *Pharmacoeconomics* 1997; **11**(6): 538–549.

89. Cohen D, Barton G. The cost to society of smoking cessation. *Thorax* 1998; **53**(Suppl 2): S38–S42.

90. Guidelines for the measurement of respiratory function. Recommendations of the British Thoracic Society and the Association of Respiratory Technicians and Physiologists. *Respir Med* 1994; **88**(3): 165–194.

91. Standardization of Spirometry, 1994 Update. American Thoracic Society. *Am J Respir Crit Care Med* 1995; **152**(3): 1107–1136.

92. Quanjer PH, Tammeling GJ, Cotes JE, Pedersen OF, Peslin R, Yernault JC. Lung volumes and forced ventilatory flows. Report Working Party Standardization of Lung Function Tests, European Community for Steel and Coal. Official Statement of the European Respiratory Society. *Eur Respir J Suppl* 1993; **16**: 5–40.

93. Standards for the diagnosis and care of patients with chronic obstructive pulmonary disease. American Thoracic Society. *Am J Respir Crit Care Med* 1995; **152**(5, Pt 2): S77–S121.

94. Traver GA, Cline MG, Burrows B. Predictors of mortality in chronic obstructive pulmonary disease. A 15-year follow-up study. *Am Rev Respir Dis* 1979; **119**(6): 895–902.

95. Chaouat A, Weitzenblum E, Kessler R, Charpentier C, Enrhart M, Schott R *et al*. A randomized trial of nocturnal oxygen therapy in chronic obstructive pulmonary disease patients. *Eur Respir J* 1999; **14**(5): 1002–1008.

96. Folgering H. Supplemental oxygen for COPD patients with nocturnal desaturations? *Eur Respir J* 1999; **14**(5): 997–999.

97. Crockett AJ, Moss JR, Cranston JM, Alpers JH. Domiciliary oxygen for chronic obstructive pulmonary disease. *Cochrane Database Syst Rev* 2000(2): CD001744.

98. Anthonisen NR, Connett JE, Kiley JP, Altose MD, Bailey WC, Buist AS *et al*. Effects of smoking intervention and the use of an inhaled anticholinergic bronchodilator on the rate of decline of FEV1. The Lung Health Study. *J Am Med Assoc* 1994; **272**(19): 1497–1505.

99. Tashkin D, Kanner R, Bailey W, Buist S, Anderson P, Nides M *et al*. Smoking cessation in patients with chronic obstructive pulmonary disease: a double-blind, placebo-controlled, randomised trial. *Lancet* 2001; **357**(9268): 1571–1575.

100. Wilcke JT. Late onset genetic disease: where ignorance is bliss, is it folly to inform relatives? *Br Med J* 1998; **317**(7160): 744–747.

101. Nuffield Council on Bioethics. *Genetic Screening – Ethical Issues*. London: Nuffield Council on Bioethics, 1993.

102. O'Donnell DE. Assessment of bronchodilator efficacy in symptomatic COPD: is spirometry useful? *Chest* 2000; **117**(2, Suppl): 42S–7S.

103. Spencer S, Calverley PM, Sherwood Burge P, Jones PW. Health status deterioration in patients with chronic obstructive pulmonary disease. *Am J Respir Crit Care Med* 2001; **163**(1): 122–128.

104. Pride NB. Smoking cessation: effects on symptoms, spirometry and future trends in COPD. *Thorax* 2001; **56**(Suppl 2): II7–II10.

105. Sethi JM, Rochester CL. Smoking and chronic obstructive pulmonary disease. *Clin Chest Med* 2000; **21**(1): 67–86, viii.

106. Scanlon PD, Connett JE, Waller LA, Altose MD, Bailey WC, Buist AS. Smoking cessation and lung function in mild-to-moderate chronic obstructive pulmonary disease. The Lung Health Study. *Am J Respir Crit Care Med* 2000; **161**(2, Pt 1): 381–390.

107. West R, McNeill A, Raw M. Smoking cessation guidelines for health professionals: an update. Health Education Authority. *Thorax* 2000; **55**(12): 987–999.

108. Lillington GA, Leonard CT, Sachs DP. Smoking cessation. Techniques and benefits. *Clin Chest Med* 2000; **21**(1): 199–208, xi.

109. Czajkowska-Malinowska M, Bednarek M, Zielinski J. Effects of repeated spirometry combined with an antismoking advice on smoking cessation rate. *Am J Respir Crit Care Med* 2001; **163**(5): A355.

110. Kerstjens HA, Brand PL, Quanjer PH, van der Bruggen-Bogaarts BA, Koeter GH, Postma DS. Variability of bronchodilator response and effects of inhaled corticosteroid treatment in obstructive airways disease. Dutch CNSLD Study Group. *Thorax* 1993; **48**(7): 722–729.

111. Calverley PM. Symptomatic bronchodilator treatment. In: Calverley PM, Pride N, editors. *Chronic Obstructive Pulmonary Disease*. London: Chapman & Hall, 1995; pp. 419–445.

112. Corris PA, Neville E, Nariman S, Gibson GJ. Dose–response study of inhaled salbutamol powder in chronic airflow obstruction. *Thorax* 1983; **38**(4): 292–296.

113. Teale C, Morrison JF, Page RL, Pearson SB. Dose response to inhaled salbutamol in chronic obstructive airways disease. *Postgrad Med J* 1991; **67**(790): 754–756.

114. Sestini P, Renzoni E, Robinson S, Poole P, Ram FS. Short-acting beta 2 agonists for stable COPD (Cochrane review). *Cochrane Database Syst Rev* 2000(3): CD001495.

115. Appleton S, Smith B, Veale A, Bara A. Long-acting beta 2-agonists for chronic obstructive pulmonary disease. *Cochrane Database Syst Rev* 2000(2): CD001104.

116. Rennard SI, Anderson W, ZuWallack R, Broughton J, Bailey W, Friedman M *et al.* Use of a long-acting inhaled beta 2-adrenergic agonist, salmeterol xinafoate, in patients with chronic obstructive pulmonary disease. *Am J Respir Crit Care Med* 2001; **163**(5): 1087–1092.

117. van Noord JA, de Munck DR, Bantje TA, Hop WC, Akveld ML, Bommer AM. Long-term treatment of chronic obstructive pulmonary disease with salmeterol and the additive effect of ipratropium. *Eur Respir J* 2000; **15**(5): 878–885.

118. Jones PW, Bosh TK. Quality of life changes in COPD patients treated with salmeterol. *Am J Respir Crit Care Med* 1997; **155**(4): 1283–1289.

119. Dahl R, Greefhorst LA, Nowak D, Nonikov V, Byrne AM, Thomson MH *et al.* Inhaled formoterol dry powder versus ipratropium bromide in chronic obstructive pulmonary disease. *Am J Respir Crit Care Med* 2001; **164**(5): 778–784.

120. Johnson M, Rennard S. Alternative mechanisms for long-acting beta (2)-adrenergic agonists in COPD. *Chest* 2001; **120**(1): 258–270.

121. Gross NJ, Co E, Skorodin MS. Cholinergic bronchomotor tone in COPD. Estimates of its amount in comparison with that in normal subjects. *Chest* 1989; **96**(5): 984–987.

122. Minette PA, Barnes PJ. Muscarinic receptor subtypes in lung. Clinical implications. *Am Rev Respir Dis* 1990; **141**(3, Pt 2): S162–S165.

123. Barnes PJ. Modulation of neurotransmission in airways. *Physiol Rev* 1992; **72**(3): 699–729.

124. Easton PA, Jadue C, Dhingra S, Anthonisen NR. A comparison of the bronchodilating effects of a beta-2 adrenergic agent (albuterol) and an anticholinergic agent (ipratropium bromide), given by aerosol alone or in sequence. *New Engl J Med* 1986; **315**(12): 735–739.

125. Braun SR, Levy SF. Comparison of ipratropium bromide and albuterol in chronic obstructive pulmonary disease: a three-center study. *Am J Med* 1991; **91**(4A): 28S–32S.

126. COMBIVENT Inhalation Aerosol Study Group. In chronic obstructive pulmonary disease, a combination of ipratropium and albuterol is more effective than either agent alone. An 85-day multicenter trial. *Chest* 1994; **105**(5): 1411–1419.

127. Martin RJ, Bartelson BL, Smith P, Hudgel DW, Lewis D, Pohl G *et al*. Effect of ipratropium bromide treatment on oxygen saturation and sleep quality in COPD. *Chest* 1999; **115**(5): 1338–1345.

128. Burge PS, Harries MG, l'Anson E. Comparison of atropine with ipratropium bromide in patients with reversible airways obstruction unresponsive to salbutamol. *Br J Dis Chest* 1980; **74**(3): 259–262.

129. Littner MR, Ilowite JS, Tashkin DP, Friedman M, Serby CW, Menjoge SS *et al*. Long-acting bronchodilation with once-daily dosing of tiotropium (Spiriva) in stable chronic obstructive pulmonary disease. *Am J Respir Crit Care Med* 2000; **161**(4, Pt 1): 1136–1142.

130. Barnes PJ. The pharmacological properties of tiotropium. *Chest* 2000; **117**(2, Suppl): 63S–6S.

131. Casaburi R, Briggs DD, Jr, Donohue JF, Serby CW, Menjoge SS, Witek TJ, Jr. The spirometric efficacy of once-daily dosing with tiotropium in stable COPD: a 13-week multicenter trial. *Chest* 2000; **118**(5): 1294–1302.

132. van Noord JA, Bantje TA, Eland ME, Korducki L, Cornelissen PJ. A randomised controlled comparison of tiotropium and ipratropium in the treatment of chronic obstructive pulmonary disease. The Dutch Tiotropium Study Group. *Thorax* 2000; **55**(4): 289–294.

133. Lightbody IM, Ingram CG, Legge JS, Johnston RN. Ipratropium bromide, salbutamol and prednisolone in bronchial asthma and chronic bronchitis. *Br J Dis Chest* 1978; **72**(3): 181–186.

134. Douglas NJ, Davidson I, Sudlow MF, Flenley DC. Bronchodilatation and the site of airway resistance in severe chronic bronchitis. *Thorax* 1979; **34**(1): 51–56.

135. Ikeda A, Nishimura K, Koyama H, Izumi T. Bronchodilating effects of combined therapy with clinical dosages of ipratropium bromide and salbutamol for stable COPD: comparison with ipratropium bromide alone. *Chest* 1995; **107**(2): 401–405.

136. Wesseling G, Mostert R, Wouters EF. A comparison of the effects of anticholinergic and beta 2-agonist and combination therapy on respiratory impedance in COPD. *Chest* 1992; **101**(1): 166–173.

137. Vassallo R, Lipsky JJ. Theophylline: recent advances in the understanding of its mode of action and uses in clinical practice. *Mayo Clin Proc* 1998; **73**(4): 346–354.

138. Halpin DMG, Hart E, Harris T, Harbour R, Rudolf M. What do general practice records tell us about the current management of COPD and the impact of the BTS COPD guidelines? *Thorax* 2000; **55**(Suppl 3): A38.

139. Murciano D, Auclair MH, Pariente R, Aubier M. A randomized, controlled trial of theophylline in patients with severe chronic obstructive pulmonary disease. *New Engl J Med* 1989; **320**(23): 1521–1525.

140. Tsukino M, Nishimura K, Ikeda A, Hajiro T, Koyama H, Izumi T. Effects of theophylline and ipratropium bromide on exercise performance in patients with stable chronic obstructive pulmonary disease. *Thorax* 1998; **53**(4): 269–273.

141. Cazzola M, Donner CF, Matera MG. Long acting beta (2) agonists and theophylline in stable chronic obstructive pulmonary disease. *Thorax* 1999; **54**(8): 730–736.

142. Karpel JP, Kotch A, Zinny M, Pesin J, Alleyne W. A comparison of inhaled ipratropium, oral theophylline plus inhaled beta-agonist, and the combination of all three in patients with COPD. *Chest* 1994; **105**(4): 1089–1094.

143. Upton RA. Pharmacokinetic interactions between theophylline and other medication (Part I). *Clin Pharmacokinet* 1991; **20**(1): 66–80.

144. Aronson JK, Hardman M, Reynolds DJ. ABC of monitoring drug therapy. Theophylline. *Br Med J* 1992; **305**(6865): 1355–1358.

145. Shannon M, Lovejoy FH, Jr. The influence of age vs peak serum concentration on life-threatening events after chronic theophylline intoxication. *Arch Intern Med* 1990; **150**(10): 2045–2048.

146. Callahan CM, Dittus RS, Katz BP. Oral corticosteroid therapy for patients with stable chronic obstructive pulmonary disease. A meta-analysis. *Ann Intern Med* 1991; **114**(3): 216–223.

147. Weir DC, Gove RI, Robertson AS, Burge PS. Corticosteroid trials in non-asthmatic chronic airflow obstruction: a comparison of oral prednisolone and inhaled beclomethasone dipropionate. *Thorax* 1990; **45**(2): 112–117.

148. Chanez P, Vignola AM, O'Shaugnessy T, Enander I, Li D, Jeffery PK *et al*. Corticosteroid reversibility in COPD is related to features of asthma. *Am J Respir Crit Care Med* 1997; **155**(5): 1529–1534.

149. Senderovitz T, Vestbo J, Frandsen J, Maltbaek N, Norgaard M, Nielsen C *et al*. Steroid reversibility test followed by inhaled budesonide or placebo in outpatients with stable chronic obstructive pulmonary disease. The Danish Society of Respiratory Medicine. *Respir Med* 1999; **93**(10): 715–718.

150. McEvoy CE, Niewoehner DE. Adverse effects of corticosteroid therapy for COPD. A critical review. *Chest* 1997; **111**(3): 732–743.

151. Vestbo J, Sorensen T, Lange P, Brix A, Torre P, Viskum K. Long-term effect of inhaled budesonide in mild and moderate chronic obstructive pulmonary disease: a randomised controlled trial. *Lancet* 1999; **353**(9167): 1819–1823.

152. Pauwels RA, Lofdahl CG, Laitinen LA, Schouten JP, Postma DS, Pride NB *et al*. Long-term treatment with inhaled budesonide in persons with mild chronic obstructive pulmonary disease who continue smoking. European Respiratory Society Study on Chronic Obstructive Pulmonary Disease. *New Engl J Med* 1999; **340**(25): 1948–1953.

153. Burge PS, Calverley PM, Jones PW, Spencer S, Anderson JA, Maslen TK. Randomised, double blind, placebo controlled study of fluticasone propionate in patients with moderate to severe chronic obstructive pulmonary disease: the ISOLDE trial. *Br Med J* 2000; **320**(7245): 1297–1303.

154. The Lung Health Study Research Group. Effect of inhaled triamcinolone on the decline in pulmonary function in chronic obstructive pulmonary disease. *New Engl J Med* 2000; **343**(26): 1902–1909.

155. Paggiaro PL, Dahle R, Bakran I, Frith L, Hollingworth K, Efthimiou J. Multicentre randomised placebo-controlled trial of inhaled fluticasone propionate in patients with chronic obstructive pulmonary disease. International COPD Study Group. *Lancet* 1998; **351**(9105): 773–780.

156. Connolly MJ. Inhaler technique of elderly patients: comparison of metered-dose inhalers and large volume spacer devices. *Age Ageing* 1995; **24**(3): 190–192.

157. Allen SC, Prior A. What determines whether an elderly patient can use a metered dose inhaler correctly? *Br J Dis Chest* 1986; **80**(1): 45–49.

158. Mestitz H, Copland JM, App B, McDonald CF. Comparison of outpatient nebulised vs metered dose inhaler terbutaline in chronic airflow obstruction. *Chest* 1989; **96**: 1237–1240.

159. Gross NJ, Petty TL, Friedman M, Skorodin MS, Silvers GW, Donohue JF. Dose response to ipratropium as a nebulized solution in patients with chronic obstructive pulmonary disease. A three-center study. *Am Rev Respir Dis* 1989; **139**(5): 1188–1191.

160. O'Driscoll BR, Kay EA, Taylor RJ, Weatherby H, Chetty MC, Bernstein A. A long-term prospective assessment of home nebulizer treatment. *Respir Med* 1992; **86**(4): 317–325.

161. Wilson RSE, Connellan SJ. Domiciliary nebulised salbutamol solution in severe chronic airway obstruction. *Thorax* 1980; **35**: 873–876.

162. Morrison JF, Jones PC, Muers MF. Assessing physiological benefit from domiciliary nebulized bronchodilators in severe airflow limitation. *Eur Respir J* 1992; **5**(4): 424–429.

163. Gunawardena KA, Smith AP, Shankleman J. A comparison of metered dose inhalers with nebulizers from the delivery of ipratropium bromide in domiciliary practice. *Br J Dis Chest* 1986; **80**(2): 170–178.

164. Jenkins SC, Heaton RW, Fulton TJ, Moxham J. Comparison of domiciliary nebulized salbutamol and salbutamol from a metered-dose inhaler in stable chronic airflow limitation. *Chest* 1987; **91**(6): 804–807.

165. O'Driscoll BR. Nebulisers for chronic obstructive pulmonary disease. *Thorax* 1997; **52**(Suppl 2): S49–S52.

166. O'Driscoll BR, Cochrane GM. Emergency use of nebulised bronchodilator drugs in British hospitals. *Thorax* 1987; **42**(7): 491–493.

167. Seemungal TA, Donaldson GC, Paul EA, Bestall JC, Jeffries DJ, Wedzicha JA. Effect of exacerbation on quality of life in patients with chronic obstructive pulmonary disease. *Am J Respir Crit Care Med* 1998; **157**(5, Pt 1): 1418–1422.

168. Seemungal TA, Donaldson GC, Bhowmik A, Jeffries DJ, Wedzicha JA. Time course and recovery of exacerbations in patients with chronic obstructive pulmonary disease. *Am J Respir Crit Care Med* 2000; **161**(5): 1608–1613.

169. Donaldson GC, Seemungal T, Jeffries DJ, Wedzicha JA. Effect of temperature on lung function and symptoms in chronic obstructive pulmonary disease. *Eur Respir J* 1999; **13**(4): 844–849.

170. Wedzicha JA. Mechanisms of exacerbations. *Novartis Found Symp* 2001; **234**: 84–93; discussion 93–103.

171. Killen J, Ellis H. Assisted discharge for patients with exacerbations of chronic obstructive pulmonary disease: safe and effective. *Thorax* 2000; **55**(11): 885.

172. Snow V, Lascher S, Mottur-Pilson C. The evidence base for management of acute exacerbations of COPD: clinical practice guideline, part 1. *Chest* 2001; **119**(4): 1185–1189.

173. Wilson R. Bacteria, antibiotics and COPD. *Eur Respir J* 2001; **17**(5): 995–1007.

174. Murphy TF, Sethi S, Niederman MS. The role of bacteria in exacerbations of COPD. A constructive view. *Chest* 2000; **118**(1): 204–209.

175. Bent S, Saint S, Vittinghoff E, Grady D. Antibiotics in acute bronchitis: a meta-analysis. *Am J Med* 1999; **107**(1): 62–67.

176. Saint S, Bent S, Vittinghoff E, Grady D. Antibiotics in chronic obstructive pulmonary disease exacerbations. A meta-analysis. *J Am Med Assoc* 1995; **273**(12): 957–960.

177. Hirschmann JV. Do bacteria cause exacerbations of COPD? *Chest* 2000; **118**(1): 193–203.

178. Anthonisen NR, Manfreda J, Warren CP, Hershfield ES, Harding GK, Nelson NA. Antibiotic therapy in exacerbations of chronic obstructive pulmonary disease. *Ann Intern Med* 1987; **106**(2): 196–204.

179. O'Driscoll BR, Taylor RJ, Horsley MG, Chambers DK, Bernstein A. Nebulised salbutamol with and without ipratropium bromide in acute airflow obstruction. *Lancet* 1989; **1**(8652): 1418–1420.

180. Thompson WH, Nielson CP, Carvalho P, Charan NB, Crowley JJ. Controlled trial of oral prednisone in outpatients with acute COPD exacerbation. *Am J Respir Crit Care Med* 1996; **154**(2, Pt 1): 407–412.

181. Niewoehner DE, Erbland ML, Deupree RH, Collins D, Gross NJ, Light RW *et al*. Effect of systemic glucocorticoids on exacerbations of chronic obstructive pulmonary disease. Department of Veterans Affairs Cooperative Study Group. *New Engl J Med* 1999; **340**(25): 1941–1947.

182. Davies L, Angus RM, Calverley PM. Oral corticosteroids in patients admitted to hospital with exacerbations of chronic obstructive pulmonary disease: a prospective randomised controlled trial. *Lancet* 1999; **354**(9177): 456–460.

183. Gravil JH, Al-Rawas OA, Cotton MM, Flanigan U, Irwin A, Stevenson RD. Home treatment of exacerbations of chronic obstructive pulmonary disease by an acute respiratory assessment service. *Lancet* 1998; **351**(9119): 1853–1855.

184. Cotton MM, Bucknall CE, Dagg KD, Johnson MK, MacGregor G, Stewart C *et al*. Early discharge for patients with exacerbations of chronic obstructive pulmonary disease: a randomised controlled trial. *Thorax* 2000; **55**(11): 902–906.

185. Skwarska E, Cohen G, Skwarski KM, Lamb C, Bushell D, Parker S *et al*. Randomised controlled trial of supported discharge in patients with exacerbations of chronic obstructive pulmonary disease. *Thorax* 2000; **55**(11): 907–912.

186. Shepperd S, Harwood D, Jenkinson C, Gray A, Vessey M, Morgan P. Randomised controlled trial comparing hospital at home care with inpatient hospital care. I: Three month follow up of health outcomes. *Br Med J* 1998; **316**(7147): 1786–1791.

187. Shepperd S, Harwood D, Gray A, Vessey M, Morgan P. Randomised controlled trial comparing hospital at home care with inpatient hospital care. II: Cost minimization analysis. *Br Med J* 1998; **316**(7147): 1791–1796.

188. Elliott MW. Noninvasive ventilation in chronic obstructive pulmonary disease. *New Engl J Med* 1995; **333**(13): 870–871.

189. Elliott MW. Non-invasive ventilation in chronic obstructive pulmonary disease. *Br J Hosp Med* 1997; **57**(3): 83–86.

190. Plant PK, Owen JL, Elliott MW. Early use of non-invasive ventilation for acute exacerbations of chronic obstructive pulmonary disease on general respiratory wards: a multicentre randomised controlled trial. *Lancet* 2000; **355**(9219): 1931–1935.

191. Greenstone M. Doxapram for ventilatory failure due to exacerbations of chronic obstructive pulmonary disease. *Cochrane Database Syst Rev* 2000(2): CD000223.

192. Corner J, Plant H, A'Hern R, Bailey C. Non-pharmacological intervention for breathlessness in lung cancer. *Palliat Med* 1996; **10**: 299–305.

193. Garner S, Eldridge F, Wagner PG, Dowell RT. Buspirone, an anxiolytic drug that stimulates respiration. *Am Rev Respir Dis* 1989; **139**: 946–950.

194. Nichol KL, Baken L, Wuorenma J, Nelson A. The health and economic benefits associated with pneumococcal vaccination of elderly persons with chronic lung disease. *Arch Intern Med* 1999; **159**(20): 2437–2442.

195. Hak E, van Essen GA, Buskens E, Stalman W, de Melker RA. Is immunising all patients with chronic lung disease in the community against influenza cost effective? Evidence from a general practice based clinical prospective cohort study in Utrecht, The Netherlands. *J Epidemiol Community Health* 1998; **52**(2): 120–125.

196. Gorse GJ, Otto EE, Daughaday CC, Newman FK, Eickhoff CS, Powers DC *et al.* Influenza virus vaccination of patients with chronic lung disease. *Chest* 1997; **112**(5): 1221–1233.

197. Chief Medical Officer. Influenza immunization programme 2001/2002. PL/CMO/2001/4. London: Department of Health, 2001.

198. Bridges CB, Fukuda K, Cox NJ, Singleton JA. Prevention and control of influenza. Recommendations of the Advisory Committee on Immunization Practices (ACIP). *MMWR Morb Mortal Wkly Rep* 2001; **50**(RR-4): 1–44.

199. Franzen D. Clinical efficacy of pneumococcal vaccination – a prospective study in patients with longstanding emphysema and/or bronchitis. *Eur J Med Res* 2000; **5**(12): 537–540.

200. Prevention of pneumococcal disease: recommendations of the Advisory Committee on Immunization Practices (ACIP). *MMWR Morb Mortal Wkly Rep* 1997; **46**(RR-8): 1–24.

201. Medical Research Council Working Party. Long term domiciliary oxygen therapy in chronic hypoxic cor pulmonale complicating chronic bronchitis and emphysema. *Lancet* 1981; **1**(8222): 681–686.

202. Nocturnal Oxygen Therapy Trial Group. Continuous or nocturnal oxygen therapy in hypoxemic chronic obstructive lung disease: a clinical trial. *Ann Intern Med* 1980; **93**(3): 391–398.

203. Calverley PM, Leggett RJ, McElderry L, Flenley DC. Cigarette smoking and secondary polycythemia in hypoxic cor pulmonale. *Am Rev Respir Dis* 1982; **125**(5): 507–510.

204. Royal College of Physicians. *Domiciliary Oxygen Therapy Services. Clinical Guidelines and Advice for Prescribers*. London: Royal College of Physicians, 1999.

205. West GA, Primeau P. Nonmedical hazards of long-term oxygen therapy. *Respir Care* 1983; **28**: 906–912.

206. Waterhouse JC, Howard P. Breathlessness and portable oxygen in chronic obstructive airways disease. *Thorax* 1983; **38**(4): 302–306.

207. Davidson AC, Leach R, George RJ, Geddes DM. Supplemental oxygen and exercise ability in chronic obstructive airways disease. *Thorax* 1988; **43**(12): 965–971.

208. Lock SH, Paul EA, Rudd RM, Wedzicha JA. Portable oxygen therapy: assessment and usage. *Respir Med* 1991; **85**(5): 407–412.

209. Garrod R, Bestall JC, Paul E, Wedzicha JA. Evaluation of pulsed dose oxygen delivery during exercise in patients with severe chronic obstructive pulmonary disease. *Thorax* 1999; **54**(3): 242–244.

210. Lock SH, Blower G, Prynne M, Wedzicha JA. Comparison of liquid and gaseous oxygen for domiciliary portable use. *Thorax* 1992; **47**(2): 98–100.

211. Lacasse Y, Wong E, Guyatt GH, King D, Cook DJ, Goldstein RS. Meta-analysis of respiratory rehabilitation in chronic obstructive pulmonary disease. *Lancet* 1996; **348**(9035): 1115–1119.

212. ATS. Pulmonary rehabilitation – 1999. *Am J Respir Crit Care Med* 1999; **159**: 1666–1682.

213. Strijbos JH, Postma DS, van Altena R, Gimeno F, Koeter GH. A comparison between an outpatient hospital-based pulmonary rehabilitation program and a home-care pulmonary rehabilitation program in patients with COPD. A follow-up of 18 months. *Chest* 1996; **109**(2): 366–372.

214. Donner CF, Muir JF. Selection criteria and programmes for pulmonary rehabilitation in COPD patients. Rehabilitation and Chronic Care Scientific Group of the European Respiratory Society. *Eur Respir J* 1997; **10**(3): 744–757.

215. Schols AM, Wouters EF. Nutritional abnormalities and supplementation in chronic obstructive pulmonary disease. *Clin Chest Med* 2000; **21**(4): 753–762.

216. Gaensler E, Cugell D, Knudson R *et al*. Surgical management of emphysema. *Clin Chest Med* 1983; **4**: 443–463.

217. Geddes DM, Davies M, Koyama H, Hansell DM, Pastorino U, Pepper JR *et al*. Effect of lung-volume-reduction surgery in patients with severe emphysema. *New Engl J Med* 2000; **343**: 239–245.

218. Cooper JD, Lefrak SS. Lung-reduction surgery: 5 years on. *Lancet* 1999; **353**(Suppl 1): 26–27.

219. Hosenpud JD, Bennett B, Keck B *et al*. The registry of the international society for heart and lung transplantation: fourteenth official report – 1997. *J Heart Lung Transplant* 1997; **16**: 691–712.

220. American Thoracic Society. International guidelines for the selection of lung transplant candidates. *Am J Respir Crit Care Med* 1998; **158**: 335–339.

221. Sundaresan RS, Shiraishi Y, Trulock EP, Manley J, Lynch J, Cooper JD *et al*. Single or bilateral lung transplantation for emphysema? *J Thorac Cardiovasc Surg* 1996; **112**(6): 1485–1494; discussion 1494–1495.

222. Meyers BF, Lynch J, Trulock E, Guthrie TJ, Cooper JD, Patterson AG. Lung transplantation: a decade of experience. *Ann Surg* 1999; **230**(3): 362–371.

223. Corris PA. Lung transplantation for chronic obstructive pulmonary disease: an exercise in quality rather than quantity? *Thorax* 1999; **54**(Suppl 2): S24–S7.

224. Stoller JK, Hoisington E, Auger G. A comparative analysis of arranging in-flight oxygen aboard commercial air carriers. *Chest* 1999; **115**(4): 991–995.

225. Johnson DC. A role for phosphodiesterase type-4 inhibitors in COPD? *Lancet* 2001; **358**(9278): 256–257.

226. Barnes PJ. Novel approaches and targets for treatment of chronic obstructive pulmonary disease. *Am J Respir Crit Care Med* 1999; **160**(5, Pt 2): S72–S9.

227. Goswami SK, Kivity S, Marom Z. Erythromycin inhibits respiratory glycoconjugate secretion from human airways *in vitro*. *Am Rev Respir Dis* 1990; **141**(1): 72–78.

Appendix 1 – Drugs

Drug	Format	Trade Name	Preparation	Strengths	Doses used in COPD	Comments	Side-effects
Short-acting beta agonists							
Salbutamol	Oral	Generic	Tablet	2 mg, 4 mg	2–4 mg 3–4 times/d	Not recommended	Tremor. Tachycardia. Hypokalaemia
		Ventmax SR	Capsule	4 mg	4–8 mg 2 times/d		
		Ventolin	Syrup	2 mg/5 ml	2–4 mg 3–4 times/d		
		Volmax	Tablet	4 mg, 8 mg	4–8 mg 2 times/d		
	Inhalation	Generic	MDI	100 mcg	200 mcg 3–4 times/d		Tremor. Tachycardia (especially with nebulized preparations)
			Nebuliser solution	1 mg/ml.	2.5–5 mg 3–4 times/d		
				2 mg/ml			
		Aerolin Autohaler	BAMDI	100 mcg	200 mcg 3–4 times/d		
		Airomir	MDI	100 mcg	200 mcg 3–4 times/d		
			BAMDI	100 mcg	200 mcg 3–4 times/d		
		Asmasal Clickhaler	DPI	95 mcg	180 mcg 3–4 times/d		
		Ventodisks	DPI	200 mcg	200 mcg 3–4 times/d		
		Ventolin	MDI	100 mcg	200 mcg 3–4 times/d		
			Accuhaler	200 mcg	200 mcg 3–4 times/d		
			BAMDI	100 mcg	200 mcg 3–4 times/d		
			Nebules	2.5 mg, 5 mg	2.5–5 mg 3–4 times/d		
			Rotacaps	200 mcg	200 mcg 3–4 times/d		

Drug	Format	Trade Name	Preparation	Strengths	Doses used in COPD	Comments	Side-effects
Terbutaline	Oral	Bricanyl	Tablet	5 mg	2.5–5 mg 3 times/d	Not recommended	Tremor, Tachycardia, Hypokalaemia
			Syrup	1.5 mg/5 ml	2.5–5 mg 3 times/d		
		Bricanyl SA	Tablet	7.5 mg	7.5 mg 2 times/d		
		Monovent	Syrup	1.5 mg/5 ml	2.5–5 mg 3 times/d		
	Inhalation	Generic	Nebulizer solution	2.5 mg/ml	5–10 mg 3–4 times/d		Tremor, Tachycardia (especially with nebulized preparations)
		Bricanyl	MDI	250 mcg	250–500 mcg 3–4 times/d		
			Turbohaler	500 mcg	500 mcg 3–4 times/d		
			Respules	2.5 mg	5–10 mg 3–4 times/d		
			Nebulizer solution	10 mg/ml	5–10 mg 3–4 times/d	Dilute with saline	
Bambuterol	Oral	Bambec	Tablet	10 mg	10–20 mg at night	Not recommended	Tremor, Tachycardia, Hypokalaemia
Fenoterol	Inhalation	Berotec	MDI	100 mcg, 200 mcg	100 mcg 1–3 times/d	Less selective than other beta agonists	Tremor, Tachycardia, Hypokalaemia
Reproterol	Inhalation	Bronchodil	MDI	500 mcg	500 mcg–1 mg 1–3 times/d		Tremor, Tachycardia, Hypokalaemia
Tulobuterol	Oral	Respacal	Tablet	2 mg	2 mg 2 times/d	Not recommended	Tremor, Tachycardia, Hypokalaemia
			Syrup	1 mg/5 ml	2 mg 2 times/d		

Drug	Format	Trade Name	Preparation	Strengths	Doses used in COPD	Comments	Side-effects
Long-acting beta agonists							
Formoterol/ Eformoterol	Inhalation	Foradil	Dry powder capsules	12 mcg	12–24 mcg 2 times/d	Rapid onset of action	Tremor, Tachycardia. Hypokalaemia
		Oxis	Turbohaler	6 mcg, 12 mcg	6–24 mcg 1–2 times/d		
Salmeterol	Inhalation	Serevent	MDI	25 mcg	50–100 mcg 2 times/d	Slow (>20 min) onset of action	Tremor, Tachycardia. Hypokalaemia. Paradoxical bronchospasms
			Accuhaler	50 mcg	50–100 mcg 2 times/d		
			Diskhaler	50 mcg	50–100 mcg 2 times/d		
Anticholinergic bronchodilators							
Ipratropium	Inhalation	Generic	Nebuliser solution	250 mcg/ml	250–500 mcg 3–4 times/d		Dry mouth, Urinary retention (rare), Blurring of vision.
		Atrovent	MDI	20 mcg, 40 mcg	40–80 mcg 3–4 times/d		
			BAMDI	20 mcg	40–80 mcg 3–4 times/d		
			DPI	40 mcg	40–80 mcg 3–4 times/d		
			Nebuliser solution	250 mcg/ml	250–500 mcg 3–4 times/d		
		Respontin	Nebuliser solution	250 mcg/ml	250–500 mcg 3–4 times/d		
Oxitropium	Inhalation	Oxivent	MDI	100 mcg	200 mcg 2–3 times/d	Slightly longer acting than ipratropium	Dry mouth, Urinary retention (rare)
		BAMDI	100mcg	200 mcg	2–3 times/d		
Tiotropium	Inhalation	Spiriva	DPI	Not yet known	18 mcg 1 time/d	Once daily. Licence expected in 2002	

Drug	Format	Trade Name	Preparation	Strengths	Doses used in COPD	Comments	Side-effects
Methylxanthines							
Theophylline	Oral	Nuelin	Tablet	125 mg	125 mg 3–4 times/d	Preparations are not interchangeable.	**Plasma levels must be monitored.** Multiple interactions with other drugs. Nausea. Tachycardia. Hypokalaemia
			Syrup	60 mg/5ml	120–240 mg 3–4 times/d		
		Neulin SA	M/R tablet	175 mg, 250 mg	175–500 mg 2 times/d		
		Lasma	M/R tablet	300 mg	300–450 mg 2 times/d		
		Slo-Phyllin	M/R capsule	60 mg, 125 mg, 250 mg	250–500 mg 2 times/d		
		Theo-Dur	M/R tablet	200 mg, 300 mg	300 mg 2 times/d		
		Uniphyllin Continus	M/R tablet	200 mg, 300 mg, 400 mg	200–400 mg 2 times/d		
Aminophylline	Oral	Generic	Tablet	100 mg	100–300 mg 3–4 times/d	Preparations are not interchangeable.	**Plasma levels must be monitored.** Multiple interactions with other drugs. Nausea. Tachycardia. Hypokalaemia
		Phyllocontin Continus	M/R tablet	225 mg, 350 mg	225–750 mg 2 times/d		

Drug	Format	Trade Name	Preparation	Strengths	Doses used in COPD	Comments	Side-effects
Corticosteroids							
Beclometasone	Inhaled	Generic	MDI	50 mcg, 100 mcg, 200 mcg	100–800 mcg 2 times/d		Oropharyngeal candidiasis, skin thinning, easy bruising osteoporosis, cateracts (N.B. side effects are dose and duration dependent)
		AeroBec	BAMDI	50 mcg, 100 mcg			
		AeroBec Forte	BAMDI	250 mcg			
		Asmabec Clickhaler	DPI	50 mcg, 100 mcg 250 mcg			
		Becodisks	DPI	100 mcg, 200 mcg, 400 mcg			
		Becotide	MDI	50 mcg, 100 mcg, 200 mcg			
			BAMDI	50 mcg, 100 mcg			
			Rotacaps	100 mcg, 200 mcg 400 mcg			
		Becloforte	MDI	250 mcg			
			BAMDI	250 mcg			
			DPI	400 mcg			
		Qvar	MDI	50 mcg, 100 mcg,			
			BAMDI	50 mcg, 100 mcg			

Drug	Format	Trade Name	Preparation	Strengths	Doses used in COPD	Comments	Side-effects
Budesonide	Inhaled	Pulmicort	MDI	50 mcg, 200 mcg,	100–800 mcg		Oropharyngeal candidiasis, skin thinning, easy bruising osteoporosis, cateracts (N.B. side-effects are dose and duration dependent)
			Turbohaler	100 mcg, 200 mcg,	2 times/d		
				400 mcg			
			Respules	250 mcg/ml	1–2 mg 2 times/d	Not recommended in COPD	
Fluticasone	Inhaled	Flixotide	MDI	25 mcg, 50 mcg,	100–1000 mcg		
				125 mcg, 250 mcg	2 times/d		
			Accuhaler	50 mcg, 100 mcg,			
				250 mcg			
			Diskhaler	50 mcg, 100 mcg,			
				250 mcg, 500 mcg			
			Nebules	250 mcg/ml	500 mcg–1 mg	Not recommended in COPD	
					2 times/d		

Drug	Format	Trade Name	Preparation	Strengths	Doses used in COPD	Comments	Side-effects
Combination Bronchodilators							
Salbutamol + Ipratropium	Inhaled	Combivent	MDI	100 mcg Salbutamol + 20 mcg Ipratropium	2 puffs 4 times/d		Tachycardia, Tremor, Dry mouth
			Nebulizer Solution	2.5 mg Salbutamol + 500 mcg Ipratropiumin 2.5 ml	1 vial 3–4 times/d		Tachycardia, Tremor, Dry mouth, Urinary retention (rare), Blurring of vision, Acute glaucoma
Fenoterol + Ipratropium	Inhaled	Duovent	MDI	100 mcg Fenoterol + 40 mcg Ipratropium	1–2 puffs 4 times/d		Tachycardia, Tremor, Dry mouth
			BAMDI	100 mcg Fenoterol + 40 mcg Ipratropium	1–2 puffs 4 times/d		
			Nebulizer Solution	1.25 mg Fenoterol + 500 mcg Ipratropium in 4 ml	1 vial 3–4 times/d		Tachycardia, Tremor, Dry mouth, Urinary retention (rare), Blurring of vision, Acute glaucoma

Combined corticosteroids and long-acting beta agonists

Drug	Format	Trade Name	Preparation	Strengths	Doses used in COPD	Comments	Side-effects
Budesonide + Eformoterol	Inhaled	Symbicort	Turbohaler	100 mcg Budesonide + 6 mcg Eformoterol 200 mcg Budesonide + 12 mcg Eformoterol	1–2 puffs 1–2 times/d	Currently no evidence on its role in COPD	Tremor, Tachycardia, Hypokalaemia. Oropharyngeal candidiasis, skin thinning, easy bruising, osteoporosis, cateracts (N.B. steroid side-effects are dose and duration dependent)
Fluticasone + Salmeterol	Inhaled	Seretide	Accuhaler	100 mcg Fluticasone + 50 mcg Salmeterol 250 mcg Fluticasone + 50 mcg Salmeterol 500 mcg Fluticasone + 50 mcg Salmeterol	1 inhalation 2 times/d	Currently no evidence on its role in COPD	Tremor, Tachycardia, Hypokalaemia. Oropharyngeal candidiasis, skin thinning, easy bruising, osteoporosis, cateracts (N.B. steroid side-effects are dose and duration dependent)

Appendix 2 – Useful Addresses and Websites

Professional societies

British Thoracic Society (www.brit-thoracic.org.uk)

BTS COPD Consortium (www.brit-thoracic.org.uk/publi/copd_publications.html)

American Thoracic Society (www.thoracic.org)

American College of Chest Physicians (www.chestnet.org)

European Respiratory Society (www.ersnet.org)

Thoracic Society of Australia & New Zealand (www.thoracic.org.au)

Canadian Thoracic Society (www.lung.ca/thorax/)

General Practice Airways Group (www.gpiag-asthma.org/GPIAG)

International Society for Heart & Lung Transplantation (www.ishlt.org)

Patient support organizations and charities

British Lung Foundation (www.lunguk.org)

American Lung Association (www.lungusa.org)

National Asthma Campaign (www.asthma.org.uk)

Alpha one (www.alpha1.org.uk)

Canadian Lung Foundation (www.lung.ca/copd/)

Other sources of information

COPD Professional (www.copdprofessional.com) (sponsored by Boehringer Ingelheim)

AZ Air (www.az-air.com) (sponsored by AstraZeneca)

Chest Net (www.chestnet.net)

Scottish Respiratory Site (www.srs.org.uk)

Colorado Health (www.coloradohealthnet.org/COPD/)

Gold Initiative (www.goldcopd.com)

Lung and Asthma Information Agency
(www.sghms.ac.uk/phs/laia/laia.htm)

National Jewish Medical & Research Centre (www.njc.org)

Mayo Clinic (www.mayohealth.org)

Training organizations

National Respiratory Training Centre (www.nrtc.org.uk)

Respiratory ERC (www.respiratoryerc.com)

Smoking cessation

ASH (www.ash.org.uk)

ASH Scotland (www.ashscotland.org.uk)

Quit (www.quit.org.uk)

NHS smoking cessation website
(www.doh.nhsweb.nhs.uk/nhssmoking cessation/)

WHO tobacco free initiative (tobacco.who.int)

Tobacco cessation guideline
(www.surgeongeneral.gov/tobacco/)

Pharmaceutical and medical gas companies and equipment manufacturers

3M (www.3M.com/us/healthcare/pharma)

AstraZeneca (www.astrazeneca.com)

BOC (www.boc.com)

Boehringer Ingelheim (www.boehringer-ingelheim.com)

Clement Clarke (www.clement-clarke.com)

Ferraris (www.ferrarismedical.com)

GlaxoSmithKline (www.gsk.com)

Micromedical (www.micromedical.co.uk)

Napp (www.napp.co.uk)

Novartis (www.novatis.com)

Vitalograph (www.vitalograph.co.uk)

Index

As COPD is the subject of this book, all index entries refer to COPD unless otherwise indicated. Page numbers followed by 'f' indicate figures; page numbers followed by 't' indicate tables. This index is in letter-by-letter order, whereby spaces and hyphens in main entries are excluded from the alphabetization process.